101 Tips™
for a
Healthy
Pregnancy
with
Diabetes

Patti B. Geil, MS, RD, FADA, CDE
Laura B. Hieronymus, MSEd, APRN, BC-ADM, CDE

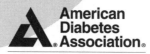

American
Diabetes
Association®

Cure • Care • Commitment℠

Director, Book Publishing, John Fedor; *Associate Director, Consumer Books,* Sherrye Landrum; *Editor,* Abe Ogden; *Associate Director, Book Production,* Peggy M. Rote; *Composition,* Circle Graphics, Inc.; *Cover Design,* Koncept, Inc.; *Printer,* Transcontinental Printing

Printed in Canada
1 3 5 7 9 10 8 6 4 2

The suggestions and information contained in this publication are generally consistent with the *Clinical Practice Recommendations* and other policies of the American Diabetes Association, but they do not represent the policy or position of the Association or any of its boards or committees. Reasonable steps have been taken to ensure the accuracy of the information presented. However, the American Diabetes Association cannot ensure the safety or efficacy of any product or service described in this publication. Individuals are advised to consult a physician or other appropriate health care professional before undertaking any diet or exercise program or taking any medication referred to in this publication. Professionals must use and apply their own professional judgment, experience, and training and should not rely solely on the information contained in this publication before prescribing any diet, exercise, or medication. The American Diabetes Association—its officers, directors, employees, volunteers, and members—assumes no responsibility or liability for personal or other injury, loss, or damage that may result from the suggestions or information in this publication.

⊚ The paper in this publication meets the requirements of the ANSI Standard Z39.48-1992 (permanence of paper).

ADA titles may be purchased for business or promotional use or for special sales. To purchase this book in large quantities, or for custom editions of this book with your logo, contact Lee Romano Sequeira, Special Sales & Promotions, at the address below, or at LRomano@diabetes.org or 703-299-2046.

American Diabetes Association
1701 North Beauregard Street
Alexandria, Virginia 22311

Library of Congress Cataloging-in-Publication Data

Geil, Patti Bazel.
    101 tips for a healthy pregnancy with diabetes / Patti Geil, Laura Hieronymus.
        p. cm.
    ISBN 1-58040-130-9 (pbk. : alk. paper)
        1. Diabetes in pregnancy. I. Title: One hundred one tips for a healthy pregnancy with diabetes. II. Hieronymus, Laura. III. Title.

RG580.D5G456 2003
618.3—dc21

2003051980

CONTENTS

▼

INTRODUCTION V

CHAPTER

1   PRIOR TO PREGNANCY 1

2   EXPECTING THE BEST: DIABETES & PREGNANCY 14

3   PREGNANCY AND NUTRITION: MORE THAN JUST
    EATING FOR TWO 22

4   MANAGING MEDICATION DURING PREGNANCY 39

5   BABY STEPS: PHYSICAL ACTIVITY DURING
    PREGNANCY 46

6   A CLOSE CHECK ON DIABETES CONTROL 58

7   PREGNANCY PEACE OF MIND 70

8   NINE MONTH SURVEILLANCE 78

9   LABOR DAY 86

10   AFTER YOUR BABY IS BORN 93

11   PREVENTING PREGNANCY: CONTROL
    BEFORE CONCEPTION 102

12   PREGNANCY POTPOURRI 108

INDEX 115

▼

To Jack, Kristen, and Rachel—
thanks for always encouraging
my great expectations!

—Patti

To my precious daughters,
Kelly and Lindsay,
whose births were blessed events
for their mother with diabetes.
And my husband, G.D.—
for always expecting the best of me!

—Laura

INTRODUCTION

▼

Of all the rights of women, the greatest is to be a mother.

Lin-Yu Tang

Less than 100 years ago, before the discovery of insulin, young women with type 1 diabetes rarely lived to reach childbearing age. Less than 30 years ago, physicians told young women with diabetes to "forget about having children"—it was considered too dangerous for both mother and baby. Today, thanks to advances in diabetes management, plus improved fetal and neonatal care, we are able to help women with diabetes experience the greatest of all rights and privileges—motherhood.

Pregnancy can be an exciting and challenging time for a woman with diabetes. Whether the diabetes is preexisting or gestational, paying close attention to blood glucose control is the key to ensuring the best health for both mother and baby. Understanding issues that are unique to women with diabetes is essential. The importance of glucose control in prepregnancy planning, during the physical and emotional changes throughout pregnancy, and even after delivery, must be a priority.

101 Tips for a Healthy Pregnancy with Diabetes is a collection of frequently asked questions by women with diabetes and those who are at risk for diabetes that are pregnant or contemplating pregnancy. As diabetes educators with professional, as well as personal experience dealing with diabetes and pregnancy, it is a privilege to share with you some of our knowledge to help answer these questions. It is our hope that all women understand just how important diabetes care and blood glucose control is for the best possible pregnancy outcome.

Chapter 1
PRIOR TO PREGNANCY

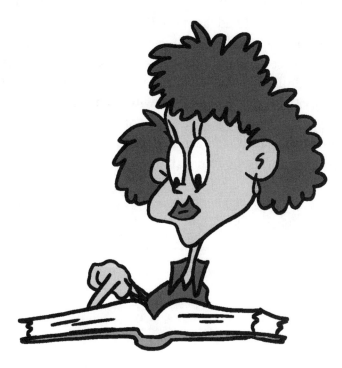

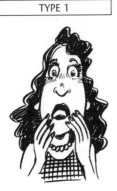

I have type 1 diabetes. Will I be able to have a baby?

▼
TIP:

Yes, with the right planning and preparation. Not too long ago, it was common for a woman with diabetes to be told she should never consider having a child. High blood glucose levels during pregnancy caused problems for the mother (worsening of diabetes complications) as well as the baby (increased risk of fetal death and birth defects). Thanks to advances in diabetes and neonatal care, a normal pregnancy and healthy baby are entirely possible *if* you keep your blood glucose levels as near normal as possible both before conception and throughout your pregnancy. If you are considering having a baby, make an appointment with your diabetes care team to discuss your pregnancy plans. Until you have achieved the best possible diabetes control and are ready to become pregnant, be sure to use a reliable form of contraception.

I have diabetes and want to become pregnant soon. My physician would like me to participate in a prepregnancy planning program. What does this involve?

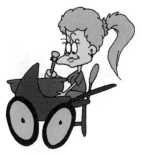

▼
TIP:

In a prepregnancy planning program your medical team will discuss with you the importance of normal blood glucose levels both before and during pregnancy, the potential risks of pregnancy for you and your baby, genetic counseling, and contraceptive advice. You should also work with a diabetes nurse educator and registered dietitian to outline a plan for achieving normal blood glucose levels. This plan will include an intensive insulin regimen, careful nutritional management, physical activity, and frequent monitoring of blood glucose levels. Research has shown that better blood glucose control before and during pregnancy lowers the risks to both mother and baby. A prepregnancy planning program is the best way to ensure that both of you are as healthy as possible.

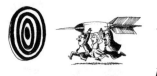

What should my target blood glucose be if I am trying to become pregnant?

TIP:

As close to normal as possible, especially before you conceive and in the first trimester of your pregnancy. The following goals for self-monitored blood glucose before conception have been recommended by the American Diabetes Association:

	Whole Blood Goals	Plasma Goals
Before meals:	70–100 mg/dl	80–110 mg/dl
2 hours after meals:	<140 mg/dl	<155 mg/dl

Adapted from "Preconception Care of Women with Diabetes," *ADA Clinical Practice Recommendations*, 2003.

Overall, your goal should be to attain the lowest A1C level you possibly can at least three months before you get pregnant, without risking excessive hypoglycemia. The A1C test measures blood glucose control over a longer period of time (about 4 months) than a fingerstick self-check of blood glucose. Research shows that if you can keep your A1C less than 1% above the normal range before your pregnancy, your chance of developing complications is dramatically reduced. The normal range is considered to be less than 6%, although this figure may vary. Near normal blood glucose levels are necessary to reduce risks and promote a healthy pregnancy outcome.

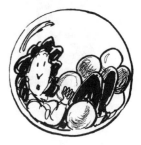

I have heard that the risk of your child having birth defects is high if you have diabetes. Is this true?

▼
TIP:

Not necessarily. This depends on your blood glucose level. If blood glucose levels are high during conception and the crucial first 8 weeks of pregnancy, the rate of birth defects and miscarriage in the first trimester can approach 65%. Common birth defects involve the heart, skeletal, and nervous systems. Since the majority of pregnancies are unplanned, it is likely that birth defects and miscarriage will occur more commonly in women with diabetes *if* they have high blood glucose when they conceive.

The good news is that research shows if you keep normal blood glucose levels before and during the early weeks of pregnancy, your risk of birth defects is similar to that of someone without diabetes. Control before conception is key!

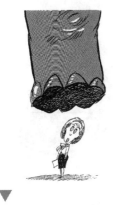

*W*ill my blood glucose control affect my ability to carry a baby to full term?

▼
TIP:

More than likely, yes. Elevated blood glucose levels put you at a higher risk for miscarriage, particularly in the first 3 months of your pregnancy. High blood glucose levels during this critical first trimester can cause the rate of miscarriage to be 30–60%, depending on how high the blood glucose is at the time of conception. High blood glucose can also cause early labor and/or birth. Babies born too early, before their lungs are fully developed, can have a serious breathing problem called respiratory distress syndrome.

Most women with diabetes have uneventful pregnancies and carry their babies to full term without any problems. But complications can occur more frequently in your baby if you have had diabetes for a long time or if you develop a condition such as toxemia, which causes high blood pressure and swelling. It's important for you to have close follow-ups during your pregnancy, preferably with a high-risk pregnancy program. A successful pregnancy with diabetes requires an investment of effort, time, and money.

I've had trouble getting pregnant and my doctor mentioned polycystic ovary syndrome (PCOS). Is this a form of diabetes?

▼
TIP:

Not necessarily, but the two are linked. Polycystic ovary syndrome, or PCOS, is the most common cause of infertility among women in the United States, affecting 5–10% of all women in the childbearing years. PCOS keeps the body from ovulating, which means eggs aren't released from the ovaries for fertilization and pregnancy cannot occur. The condition is linked with insulin resistance, a condition in which the body resists the action of the hormone insulin, as well as obesity and excessive male hormones.

Because it is linked to insulin resistance, PCOS is also associated with type 2 diabetes. Fifty percent of women with type 2 diabetes develop PCOS and 30% of obese women with PCOS develop glucose intolerance or type 2 diabetes by age 40. Women with type 2 diabetes and/or PCOS are also more susceptible to cardiovascular disease.

If you are diagnosed with PCOS, an oral contraceptive or a medication such as metformin may be prescribed to reduce insulin resistance. Healthy eating and physical activity for weight control should also be part of a program intended to restore your fertility. Should you become pregnant, you may be at risk for gestational diabetes due to your underlying insulin resistance and the added insulin resistance that normally occurs with pregnancy, especially after the 16th week of your pregnancy.

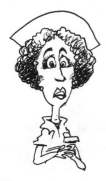

*S*ix months ago I was told I have pre-
diabetes. Is it okay for me to have a
baby?

▼
TIP:

Yes, but once again, only if you take the appropriate precautions.
Pre-diabetes, formerly referred to as *impaired glucose
tolerance*, means that your blood glucose levels are above the normal range, but not high enough for you to be diagnosed with type 2
diabetes. Most people with pre-diabetes are well on their way to
diabetes unless lifestyle changes, such as increased physical activity
and improved nutrition, are made.

If you have pre-diabetes and you want to become pregnant, prepregnancy planning is essential. Work with your health care team to
determine your overall health and to stay up to date on your blood
glucose levels. Working with a registered dietitian (RD) is helpful as
well. An RD can establish nutrition needs, a healthy body weight,
and provide physical activity tips that will benefit your overall
health and work to normalize your blood glucose levels prior to
conception.

Because insulin resistance occurs normally in pregnancy due to
hormonal changes, you will need medical guidance from someone
with expertise in diabetes and pregnancy to help you manage your
blood glucose levels throughout your pregnancy.

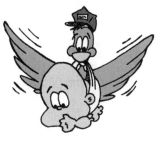

I am 28 years old and have had type 1 diabetes since I was 13. Is it okay for me to have a baby?

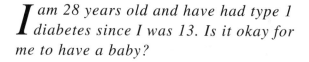

▼

TIP:

Yes, but be sure to meet with your physician to discuss the issue beforehand. Your physician should discuss the following with you:

■ current contraception methods, to ensure you attain normal blood glucose levels before you get pregnant
■ risks of pregnancy, to both you and your child
■ the importance of maintaining normal blood glucose levels for several months prior to pregnancy. Studies have shown that intensive management of diabetes and normal blood glucose levels before pregnancy can lower the risk of complications to nondiabetes levels
■ genetic counseling, which can determine your baby's risk of developing diabetes. Your age at the time of pregnancy can influence this risk. If you have type 1 and are less than 25 when you conceive, the chance of your baby developing type 1 diabetes is about 4%; if you're older than 25 years, the chance decreases to about 1%.
■ any complications you may have. Having complications does not automatically mean you can't have a child, but if you do have complications, understanding how they will affect your pregnancy and how your pregnancy will affect your complications is essential.
■ your level of commitment. Having diabetes means pregnancy will be a lot more work. If you're not committed to an increased level of medical and obstetric supervision, the ability and willingness to perform frequent blood glucose testing, and undergoing prompt follow-ups to treatment plans, you may not be ready for pregnancy. If, however, you feel like you can meet these extra demands, a happy and healthy pregnancy may be in your future.

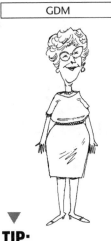

*M*y mother has diabetes. Does this increase my risk of developing gestational diabetes?

TIP:

Yes. Women who have a strong family history of diabetes are at a higher risk for developing gestational diabetes, or GDM (see page 16). GDM first occurs during pregnancy and usually disappears after the birth of the baby. Almost 7% of all pregnancies are affected by GDM and your chances of developing it increase if you:

- have a family history of diabetes
- have previously had a very large baby or stillbirth
- are overweight
- had an earlier pregnancy with GDM
- are older than 25 years of age

Because of your high-risk status, your physician should immediately evaluate you for GDM with glucose testing if you do become pregnant. If there's no sign of GDM at your first screening, you should be checked again 24–28 weeks into your pregnancy, which is when GDM is most often detected.

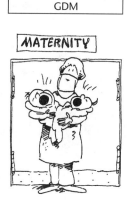

I *had gestational diabetes with my last pregnancy. Will I have it again?*

▼
TIP:

Although any pregnant woman can develop gestational diabetes (GDM), because of your previous history of GDM, you are more likely to develop it than others. Gestational diabetes occurs when the pregnancy hormones produced by your placenta cause your body to become resistant to insulin. You may become unable to produce enough insulin to meet your body's needs, so your blood glucose levels slowly rise and reach levels above normal by about 24–28 weeks into your pregnancy. At this point, a healthy meal plan, physical activity, and maybe even insulin injections will be needed to keep blood glucose levels in control and prevent complications in your baby.

If you do become pregnant, your physician should evaluate you for GDM with blood glucose testing as soon as possible. It may be necessary to repeat the blood glucose screening as your pregnancy progresses, particularly between 24–28 weeks.

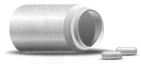

I've been told I need to take a prenatal vitamin before trying to become pregnant. Why?

▼
TIP:

You want the best possible nutritional status before, during, and after pregnancy for your health and for the health of your child. Folic acid is especially important before pregnancy. It reduces the risk of certain birth defects, such as cleft palate and spina bifida. All women of childbearing age, whether they have diabetes or not, are advised to get 400 mcg of folic acid per day from fortified foods, supplements, or a combination of both for a period of time before becoming pregnant.

Iron is another important nutrient. If a woman has iron-deficiency anemia when she becomes pregnant, it may be difficult to build up her iron stores during pregnancy.

Eating whole grains, vegetables, and fruits as part of healthy daily eating is the best guarantee that you will have all the nutrients you need. Women most likely to benefit from taking supplements are those who don't eat healthfully, are underweight or constantly trying to lose weight, or abuse alcohol or drugs. Seek professional nutrition guidance so you get the vitamins and minerals you need and don't get too much of the ones you don't need.

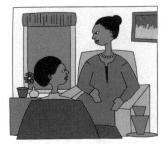

I have had type 1 diabetes for 14 years. My diabetes educator suggested that I begin using an insulin pump before I try to become pregnant. Why?

▼
TIP:

Maintaining as near-to-normal blood glucose levels as possible for at least 3 months before conception—and throughout pregnancy—lowers the risk of complications for both you and your baby. Women with type 1 diabetes who are planning to get pregnant often watch their meal plan more closely, check blood glucose levels more often, and take up to 4 injections daily or use an insulin pump. An insulin pump allows you to get near-normal glucose levels by delivering insulin as needed to match up with the food you eat, the action of pregnancy hormones, and blood glucose levels that fluctuate more as pregnancy progresses. You could wait to begin insulin pump therapy until after you become pregnant, but using it for glucose control before pregnancy gives you time to learn how to use it well. With an insulin pump, you need to be committed to doing blood checks often, counting carbs, and learning to adjust your insulin dose. To succeed, you need to be motivated and to have strong support at home and the doctor's office.

Chapter 2
EXPECTING THE BEST
Diabetes & Pregnancy

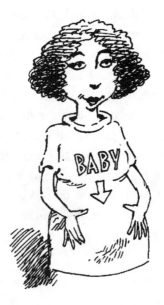

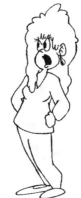

I've heard that pregnancy hormones
affect blood sugar levels. Is this true?

▼

TIP:

Yes. The placenta is a flat, circular organ that links the unborn
baby to the mother's uterus during pregnancy. It produces *contrainsulin* hormones, such as human placental lactogen, prolactin,
estrogen, and progesterone. The production of these hormones,
along with increased levels of cortisol, can affect your body's sensitivity to insulin, whether it is insulin produced by your own body,
insulin injected by syringe or pen, *or* insulin infused by an insulin
pump. Although these hormones are essential to a healthy pregnancy, this hormonal "aggravation," along with the weight you'll
gain as your pregnancy progresses, can contribute to a rise in blood
glucose levels, particularly after the 18th week of your pregnancy.

The best way to ensure your glucose levels are under control is
to know where your glucose levels are at all times. Frequent self-
glucose monitoring (up to 8 times a day when you are pregnant) can
help identify changes in blood glucose levels. This will help you and
your diabetes health team make the necessary changes for the best
blood glucose control throughout your pregnancy.

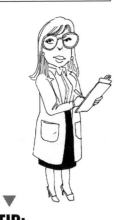

I am pregnant and my doctor says I am at risk for gestational diabetes. What does that mean?

▼
TIP:

Gestational diabetes mellitus, or GDM, means your blood glucose levels are higher than normal for a pregnant woman. Unless you already have diabetes (in which case there's no need to screen for diabetes—you already know), your obstetrician should consider whether or not you need a GDM screening based on your risk for developing GDM.

Low Risk (probably will not be screened for GDM):
- Member of an ethnic group with low prevalence of GDM
- No known diabetes in first-degree relatives
- Younger than 25 years old
- Weight normal before pregnancy
- No history of abnormal glucose metabolism
- No history of poor pregnancy outcome

Average Risk (usually screened for GDM at 24–28 weeks):
- Any woman who does not meet all of the "Low Risk" conditions but is not considered "High Risk"

High Risk (should be screened for GDM early in pregnancy and again at 24–28 weeks):
- Marked obesity, strong family history of type 2 diabetes, personal history of GDM, glucose intolerance, or glucose present in the urine
- Various ethnic groups with a high prevalence of GDM (includes Native American, African American, and Hispanic women)

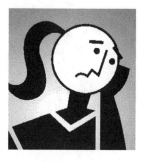

*M*y doctor says I need to be screened for gestational diabetes. What does that involve?

▼
TIP:

Generally, the screening for GDM goes as follows:

Initial Screening
- Fasting is not required
- You will take 50 grams of a glucose solution
- A laboratory will analyze your glucose reading
- If your glucose reading is higher than 130 mg/dl, an oral glucose tolerance test (GTT) is recommended.

Diagnosis and GTT
- Fasting is required
- A laboratory will analyze your fasting glucose reading
- You will then take 100 grams of a glucose solution (sometimes 75 grams)
- A laboratory will analyze your glucose levels at 1, 2, and 3 hours after you take the glucose solution (or just 1 and 2 hours after taking 75 grams of solution)

Sometimes this procedure will be modified. In high-risk populations, a health care professional might skip the initial screening and go straight to the GTT, usually because it's less expensive. Some medical professionals suggest an GTT only if your initial screening is higher than 140 mg/dl, instead of the 130 mg/dl level listed above. It's important to remember that all glucose readings should come from laboratory analysis. Readings from fingerstick methods are not good enough to make a diagnosis.

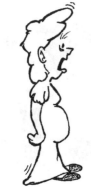

I've just found out I have gestational diabetes and I'm worried about birth defects. What are the chances that my baby will have a birth defect?

TIP:

This depends. Birth defects have been linked to poor blood glucose control in a number of studies. Because the development of vital organs (such as the spine, heart, and brain) occurs mostly by the 8th week of pregnancy, it is essential that women with pre-existing diabetes have near-normal blood glucose control before conception to decrease the risk of birth defects. Gestational diabetes (GDM) makes things a little tricky, however, since it isn't diagnosed until pregnancy has already begun. Although GDM is typically diagnosed during the late 2nd or early 3rd trimester of the pregnancy, it is possible that blood glucose levels may have been high earlier in the pregnancy. If blood sugar levels were normal as vital organs were developing, then the risk of birth defects would be similar to any pregnant woman without diabetes—about 3–6%. However, if glucose levels were less than optimal during this period, then the risk for birth defects may be increased. It's always a good idea to discuss any concerns you have about birth defects with your health care team.

I *have been experiencing hypoglycemia*
without realizing it while I am
pregnant. Is this common?

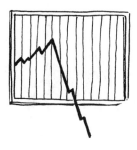

▼
TIP:

M any women experience "hypoglycemia unawareness" during pregnancy, although you do not have to be pregnant for this to happen. This condition generally only affects women who are using insulin to control their diabetes, since they are the ones at risk for hypoglycemia (low blood sugar). Hypoglycemia unawareness can be especially common during pregnancy because hypoglycemia can be more common. When you're pregnant, the recommended goals for glucose control are lower than goals for the nonpregnant person with diabetes. Your brain may get comfortable with lower levels of blood glucose and be less sensitive to the warning signs you get when you're "too low" (usually 60 mg/dl or less). In addition, there's also the possibility that the fetus can deplete carbohydrate and calorie stores in your blood, which can also cause hypo-glycemia.

Work with your diabetes health care team to lower your risk of hypoglycemia. Checking your blood glucose up to 8 times a day is often recommended. This can help you identify blood glucose patterns, as well as "at-risk" times for hypoglycemia. Having a "Glucagon Emergency Kit" (see page 45) on hand is also an important part of your diabetes plan. Your health care team can provide a prescription for the kit and show you how it's used.

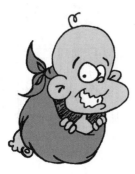

Will severe hypoglycemia affect my baby?

▼
TIP:

There is very little data that supports a direct connection between hypoglycemia (low blood sugar) and fetal danger. However, this does not mean that hypoglycemia is not dangerous. Symptoms of severe hypoglycemia, which include confused or hostile states of mind, lack of coordination, fatigue, and even passing out, can increase the risk of an accident, which may be harmful to both you and the fetus.

Hypoglycemia is a risk for all women with diabetes who take insulin. Hypoglycemia unawareness, a condition where you do not recognize low blood glucose, may also be exaggerated during pregnancy, especially in women with type 1 diabetes (see page 19). Women with diabetes who are pregnant—especially those on insulin therapy—are asked to monitor their blood glucose levels up to 8 times daily. You are advised to treat blood glucose levels of 60 mg/dl or below whether you have symptoms or not. You should check blood glucose levels before you drive, as well.

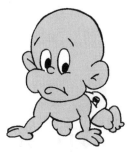

*M*y doctor says, based on the results of my amniocentesis, I need to take steroid injections. She also mentioned something about respiratory distress syndrome. What does all of that mean?

▼
TIP:

An *amniocentesis* is a procedure in which your health care pro-fessional (usually your obstetrician or perinatologist) will take a sample of amniotic fluid from your uterus. The sample is then ana-lyzed to determine if your fetus is at risk for respiratory distress syndrome, a condition that affects your newborn baby's ability to breathe. There are studies that indicate that the risk of respiratory distress syndrome is greater in infants whose mothers have diabetes. Because of this risk, women with diabetes will usually have at least one amniocentesis before delivery to determine if the fetus' lungs are mature. If the results show immature fetal lungs, then a steroid, such as dexamethasone, is usually given by injection on 2 consecu-tive days to help the fetal lungs mature. The procedure should be monitored very closely since dexamethasone can cause hyper-glycemia (high blood sugar). You may need to change your insulin dosages during the course of the therapy to counteract the steroids. If time permits, your physician may repeat the amniocentesis at a later date before starting any steroid therapy.

Chapter 3
PREGNANCY AND NUTRITION
More than Just Eating for Two

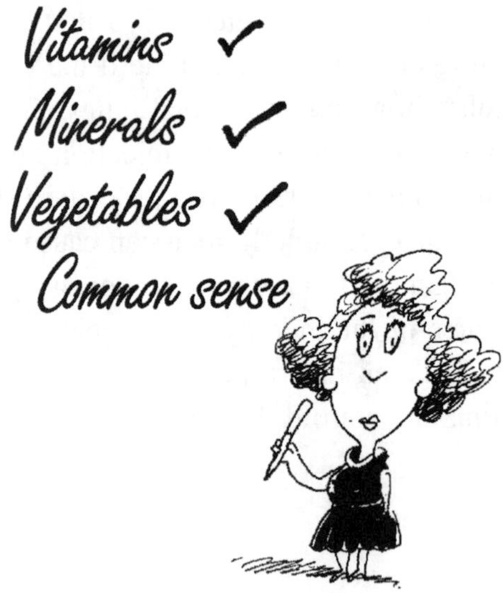

Vitamins ✓
Minerals ✓
Vegetables ✓
Common sense

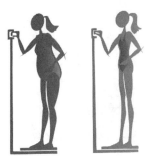

*H*ow much weight should I gain
during my pregnancy?

▼
TIP:

A s a woman with diabetes, there are no special issues regarding
your weight gain, as long as you are eating a nutritionally
healthy diet and your blood glucose levels are within the recommended ranges. Weight gain during pregnancy is normal, even necessary for successful outcomes, yet many women (even those without
diabetes) worry about pregnancy-related weight gain. Basically, the
amount of weight you should gain is based on your body mass index
(BMI) and your weight before pregnancy. Your BMI is a combination
of weight and height. To determine your BMI, multiply your prepregnancy weight by 705, divide this number by your height in inches,
and then divide this number by your height again. Or just check a
BMI chart.

The basic guidelines for pregnancy-related weight gain are as follows:

BMI	Recommended Weight Gain
Less than 19.8	28–40 pounds
19.8–26	25–35 pounds
26.1–29	15–25 pounds
More than 29	15 pounds
Exceptions	
Twin pregnancy	34–45 pounds
Triplet pregnancy	About 50 pounds

As always, check with your diabetes care team for the amount of
weight gain that's right for you.

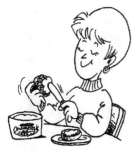

I have type 2 diabetes and was quite overweight when I became pregnant. Should I try to lose a few pounds for a healthier pregnancy?

▼
TIP:

No. It's true that women who are overweight during pregnancy may experience more medical problems, such as hypertension (high blood pressure) and preeclampsia (hypertension and swelling caused by pregnancy). However, pregnancy is not the time to lose weight. Cutting down on calories can cause your body to burn fat stores, resulting in ketones, which could be harmful to your baby. Although you shouldn't be dieting, you should limit your weight gain to about 15 pounds while you are pregnant. Hold your weight gain steady and vow to yourself that you'll drop the pounds after the baby is born.

*M*y obstetrician says I'm gaining
weight too quickly. Is there an ideal
rate of weight gain during pregnancy?

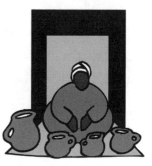

▼
TIP:

There is no "ideal" formula for weight gain. However, weight gain should be gradual and follow a predictable pattern. During the 1st trimester, you should gain 2–5 pounds *total*. Almost all of this weight is gained as your uterus and breasts enlarge, your blood volume expands, and the placenta and amniotic fluid is formed. During the 2nd and 3rd trimesters, a healthy rate of weight gain is 1/2 to 1 pound a week. The last trimester is when the baby is growing the most. If your weight gain slows during the last trimester there's a higher risk you'll deliver the baby before it is due.

Throughout your pregnancy, your goal should be to keep your weight gain steady and your blood glucose under control. If you notice any sudden weight gain or loss during your pregnancy, check with your health team to rule out any serious problems. A registered dietitian with expertise in pregnancy and diabetes can work with you to design a healthy eating plan for you during pregnancy.

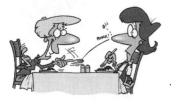

I've often heard that pregnant women are eating for two. How much extra food should I be eating?

▼
TIP:

Eating for two doesn't mean you should be eating twice as many calories each day! Generally, the recommended calorie intake for an active pregnant woman is 2400–2800 calories—about 300 more calories a day than usual. However, because your baby's health is so closely linked to your own, you should pack as much nutrition as you can into each meal. It's important to eat a healthy variety of foods from each food group. The table below is based on the Diabetes Food Pyramid. It shows the different food groups and example servings from each. Talk with your dietitian about how many servings from each food group you should eat to meet your daily calorie goals. Foods with an * are sources of carbohydrate; your intake of these should be based on your blood glucose levels.

Food Group	Examples of a Serving
*Grains, Beans, and Starchy Vegetables	1 slice of bread 1/3 cup cooked beans 1/2 cup cooked cereal
*Vegetables	1 cup raw vegetables 1/2 cup cooked vegetables 1/2 cup vegetable juice
*Fruits	1 small apple 1/2 medium banana 1/2 cup apple juice
*Milk	1 cup milk 1 cup yogurt
Meat and Others	2–3 ounces of cooked lean meat, poultry, or fish 1/2 cup tofu
*Fats and Sweets	Variable serving sizes; use with caution
Alcohol	Do not drink alcohol while you are pregnant!

A re there any vitamin supplements I should be taking while I'm pregnant?

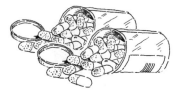

▼
TIP:

M aybe. If you make healthy food choices from a variety of food groups, you will generally receive all the vitamins and minerals you need. However, certain vitamins and minerals may require special attention.

- **Folic Acid**—You should consume at least 400 micrograms of folic acid every day, whether it is from foods, supplements, or both. Folic acid can be found in legumes, green leafy vegetables, liver, citrus fruits and juices, and whole-wheat bread.
- **Iron**—A routine, low-dose iron supplement of 30 milligrams a day is recommended for all pregnant women. You can also find iron in lean red meat, fish, poultry, dried fruits, and iron-fortified cereals.
- **Zinc and Copper**—Iron can interfere with the absorption of other minerals, so if you are taking an iron supplement you should also be taking 15 milligrams of zinc and 2 milligrams of copper daily. You can find these minerals in most prenatal vitamin and mineral supplements.
- **Calcium**—If you are 14–18 years old, you should be getting at least 1300 milligrams of calcium daily; if you're 19–50 years old, you should be getting 1000 milligrams. Dairy products are the best source of calcium.

There are some specific pregnancy cases where it is highly recommended you take a supplement. If you smoke or abuse drugs or alcohol, have iron deficiency anemia, rarely or never eat meat, or are pregnant with more than one fetus, then you should probably be taking a supplement. Talk with your diabetes care team to see which minerals or vitamins you require during pregnancy.

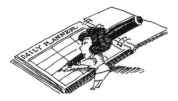

*C*an I use carbohydrate counting to plan my meals while I'm pregnant?

▼
TIP:

Yes, carbohydrate counting is an excellent way to plan your meals while you are pregnant. Carbohydrate has the biggest effect on your after-meal blood glucose levels, so an adequate and consistent level of carbohydrate is an important factor in keeping your blood glucose levels under control and your pregnancy healthy. Carbohydrates are found in grains, vegetables, fruit, milk, and sweets.

Work with a registered dietitian (RD) to plan a diet that has the correct amount of carbohydrate for your pregnancy. Generally, 40–45% of your calories should come from carbohydrate, although this can vary from person to person. An RD can figure out a more specific number for you and your needs. An RD can also help you learn more about portion size, which is critical to carbohydrate counting. If you are taking insulin, whether through injections or through a pump, you'll need to know how much carbohydrate you are eating to adjust your insulin doses. If you do intend to plan your meals with carbohydrate counting, remember that self-monitoring of blood glucose levels is very important.

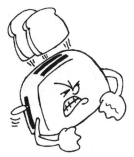

*M*y registered dietitian told me to
limit the amount of carbohydrate
I'm eating in the morning. Why?

▼
TIP:

Because pregnant women don't handle carbohydrate as well in
the morning as they do at other times of the day. This is due to
the increase of pregnancy hormone levels in the morning, which
work against insulin. Basically, pregnant women tend to be more
glucose intolerant in the morning. Many meal plans for pregnant
women will have 30 grams of carbohydrate for breakfast—equal to
1 slice of toast and 1 cup of milk (8 ounces). If this isn't satisfying
your hunger, try adding protein to your morning meal. Protein
doesn't affect your after-meal glucose levels that much, and it is
filling.

Check your blood glucose levels often. If your after-breakfast
glucose levels are within target range, you may be able to add a
small amount of carbohydrate back to your breakfast. If your blood
glucose levels are high, you might need to reduce your morning
carbohydrate intake or begin doing some moderate exercise after
breakfast.

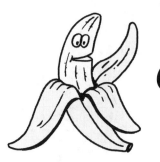

*C*an I have snacks between meals?

▼
TIP:

O f course. Snacks provide a constant source of nutrition for your growing baby and help you avoid extreme changes in blood glucose levels. In addition, smaller and more frequent meals and snacks can help prevent the heartburn and nausea that usually go hand in hand with pregnancy.

Unfortunately, many pregnant women with diabetes skip meals or snacks, thinking this will help keep their blood glucose under control. Do not do this! Going long periods of time without food can cause your body to burn fat, which leads to the presence of ketones in your bloodstream and "starvation ketosis." This can have a very negative impact on your baby's brain development. Your baby also requires a steady source of glucose 24 hours a day, not just while you're awake. This makes a bedtime snack very important.

Check your blood glucose often throughout the day and work with your registered dietitian to develop a meal plan that is right for you. Most pregnant women find that a meal plan of 3 meals a day with 3 between-meal snacks is best. Snacks that contain protein, such as peanut butter or low-fat cheese, can help satisfy hunger without having a big impact on blood glucose levels.

*I*s it safe for me to use artificial
sweeteners while I'm pregnant?

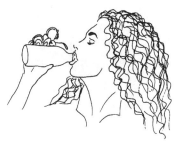

▼
TIP:

For the most part. The effects of artificial sweeteners on pregnancy have been well studied. Currently, the Food and Drug Administration (FDA) has approved 5 nonnutritive, artificial sweeteners as being safe for use during pregnancy. But keep the following in mind.

- **Saccharin** crosses the placenta and can remain in fetal tissues, although it does not appear to be harmful. You should still probably avoid this sweetener.
- **Acesulfame-K** also crosses the placenta, but once again, there doesn't appear to be any harmful side effects. There are no specific recommendations for using this sweetener during pregnancy.
- **Aspartame** must be present in very large amounts to cross the placenta, but it appears to be safe if you keep your intake within the FDA guidelines. Women with phenylketonuria should use aspartame with caution.
- **Sucralose** appears to be a safe sweetener during pregnancy. The FDA has concluded that sucralose poses no reproductive risk.
- **Neotame** is the most recent FDA-approved sweetener. Research shows that it is safe for use in pregnant and breastfeeding women.

Nutritive sweeteners, such as fructose and sorbitol, contain carbohydrate that must be counted in your meal plan. Remember to read your food labels closely and talk with your medical team about your use of sweeteners.

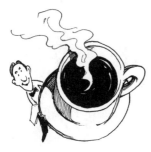

*D*o I need to limit caffeine intake while I'm pregnant?

▼
TIP:

It might not be a bad idea. Caffeine can cross the placenta and affect your baby's heart rate and breathing, although no studies in humans have found that caffeine is linked with birth defects. However, most health care professionals recommend that pregnant women keep their caffeine intake to about 300 milligrams a day. The following chart lists the amount of caffeine found in common foods and beverages.

Beverage	Serving Size	Amount of Caffeine
Percolated coffee	5 ounces	85 mg
Instant coffee	5 ounces	60 mg
Espresso	1 ounce	40 mg
Leaf/bag tea	5 ounces	30 mg
Soda/cola beverage	12 ounces	36 mg

Discuss your use of caffeine with your health care team and learn what they recommend for you and your situation.

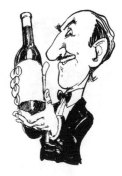

Will it hurt the baby if I have an occasional alcoholic drink while I'm pregnant?

▼
TIP:

Yes! If you are pregnant or may become pregnant, you should not drink alcohol. Period. Alcohol crosses the placenta, so your baby will be exposed to any alcohol you drink. Heavy drinking during pregnancy seriously increases the risk of mental retardation, learning disabilities, and major birth defects, a condition known as *fetal alcohol syndrome*. Even moderate drinking (no more than 1 serving of alcohol a day) has been linked to lower fertility rates and fetal growth problems. Beer, wine, and other alcoholic beverages carry a warning label about the dangers of drinking while pregnant. So save the champagne to celebrate after your baby is born!

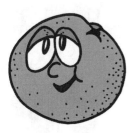

*F*ruit seems to help the constipation
I've had since becoming pregnant,
but it has a lot of carbohydrate. Is there
something else I should be using?

▼ TIP:

Not necessarily. Constipation is a normal part of pregnancy. Pregnancy hormones tend to relax digestive muscles and slow down the digestion process. Iron supplements can also lead to constipation. If fruits tend to relieve your constipation troubles, then by all means, keep eating fruit. Just be sure to count the carbohydrate as part of your overall meal plan. Fruit probably helps because it has fiber and fiber-rich foods, such as legumes, whole grains, bran, and vegetables can help aid in digestion. All of these foods contain carbohydrate. If you're looking for a noncarbohydrate approach, try drinking 8–12 cups of water a day and getting moderate daily exercise. These activities can help keep you regular. If the problem persists, check with your health care team for other options.

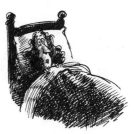

I *have suffered from morning sickness*
throughout my pregnancy. Would it be
safe for me to try an herbal remedy?

▼
TIP:

No. Until the safety of herbal remedies with pregnancy is proven, it's best to avoid using them. There have been very few scientific studies done looking at the safety of alternative therapies. While herbal remedies sound safe because they are "natural," some may cause severe side effects, such as increased bleeding.

The bigger concern here is the effect morning sickness can have on your diabetes. Morning sickness is a very normal part of pregnancy, though its causes are still not understood. We do know that it tends to be worse when your stomach is empty, so you may find relief by just eating smaller meals more frequently, avoiding offensive odors, drinking more water, and getting more fresh air. Depending on how well you tolerate carbohydrate, your health care team may suggest you eat a carbohydrate food, such as rice cakes or saltines, before getting out of bed in the morning. These snacks will also help prevent ketonuria, which can make morning sickness worse.

Nausea can also be a sign of hypoglycemia, and hypoglycemia can make nausea worse, so be prepared to check your blood glucose often. If you're taking insulin, you may need to adjust your dosage on a meal-to-meal basis while you figure out which foods you can stomach. If your morning sickness and vomiting become severe, your medical team may suggest you be hospitalized to avoid dehydration and electrolyte imbalances.

There is a silver lining to all of this, however. Morning sickness usually disappears after the 3rd month of pregnancy *and* women who have morning sickness are less likely to have a miscarriage or premature birth.

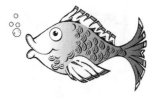

My obstetrician told me to avoid certain types of fish while I'm pregnant. Why?

▼
TIP:

B ecause some types of fish contain methyl mercury, which can be harmful to developing nervous systems. Your obstetrician's worries are backed by the Food and Drug Administration (FDA), which has released information on the dangers of eating certain types of fish while you are pregnant, planning to become pregnant, or nursing. Methyl mercury occurs naturally in the environment, but is also a by-product of industrial pollution. Generally, methyl mercury is found in large, long-lived fish, such as the shark, swordfish, king mackerel, and tilefish. These fish should be avoided while you are pregnant. It is probably safe to eat up to 12 ounces of cooked fish per week, so long as they are smaller types of fish. You may want to contact your local health department to find out if there are any special warnings about toxins in fish caught or sold in your area.

I heard a news report about something called "listeriosis" and how it is especially dangerous for pregnant women. What is it and should I be worried?

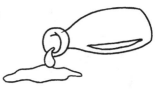

▼
TIP:

L isteriosis is a food-borne illness caused by the bacteria *listeria monocytogenes* and is especially dangerous for pregnant women and their unborn babies. It can cause premature delivery, miscarriage, fetal death, and severe illness or death in a newborn who has been infected. Pregnant women and their unborn babies are 20 times more likely than other healthy adults to get listeriosis. With that in mind, it's best to be cautious. To reduce your risk of getting listeriosis, avoid foods that are more likely to be carrying the bacterium, such as soft cheeses (feta, Brie, Camembert), unpasteurized milk, hot dogs, lunch meats, and deli meats. Signs of the illness include flu-like symptoms and problems with the nervous system, such as headache, stiff neck, and confusion. Antibiotics are the recommended treatment. If you think you have listeriosis, talk with your medical team immediately. A blood test can confirm whether or not you have the illness.

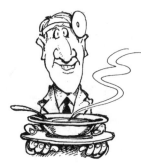

*W*hat is a registered dietitian and
where can I find one?

▼
TIP:

A registered dietitian (RD) is the nutrition expert on your diabetes
care team, the one who will help you develop a meal plan
specifically tailored to your needs as a pregnant woman with diabetes. An RD with experience in pregnancy and diabetes will be
especially helpful. Your primary doctor may recommend an RD, or
you may find one at a local hospital, outpatient clinic, or health
department. The following resources may also be helpful.

- To find a registered dietitian in your area, call the American
  Dietetic Association at 1-800-877-1600, or visit their website at
  www.eatright.org.
- To find a diabetes education program that has been approved by
  the American Diabetes Association, call 1-800-342-2383, or visit
  their website at *www.diabetes.org*.
- To find a diabetes educator, call the American Association of
  Diabetes Educators at 1-800-832-6874, or visit their website at
  www.aadenet.org.

Chapter 4
MANAGING MEDICATION DURING PREGNANCY

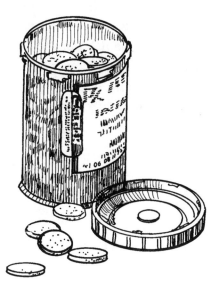

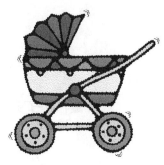

*W*ill insulin therapy have a negative effect on my baby?

▼
TIP:

No. Insulin therapy has been used safely to reach and/or maintain the best possible glucose control in pregnancy for years. We know that glucose crosses the placenta to the fetus. The effects of hyperglycemia (high blood glucose) during pregnancy are well documented and include a higher incidence of birth defects, increased rate of miscarriage, and macrosomia (a larger than normal fetus). Insulin therapy, whether injected or infused through an insulin pump, has an essential role in keeping your glucose levels under control for you and your baby. Published studies have confirmed that good blood glucose levels lower the risks to the fetus throughout your pregnancy. Insulin is a vital part of a healthy pregnancy for a woman with high blood glucose.

I have gestational diabetes and my doctor says I need to take insulin. My mother takes pills for her diabetes. Why can't I?

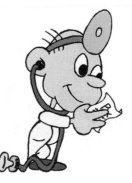

▼
TIP:

B ecause you are pregnant and your mother is not (we're assuming). Oral medications can often be used to treat type 2 diabetes, depending on an individual's needs. However, oral glucose lowering agents have generally not been recommended *during pregnancy*. If your blood glucose control is not meeting the recommended goals for diabetes and pregnancy, the medication of choice is insulin therapy. Insulin therapy should be recommended if blood glucose levels exceed the following:

	Whole Blood Goals	**Plasma Goals**
Fasting	≤95 mg/dl	≤105 mg/dl
1 hour post meal	≤140 mg/dl	≤155 mg/dl
2 hours post meal	≤120 mg/dl	≤130 mg/dl

Adapted from "Gestational Diabetes Mellitus," *ADA Clinical Practice Recommendations,* 2003.

Most health care professionals recommend insulin therapy if blood glucose levels fall outside the above ranges within a 1–2 week period. The type of insulin therapy used during pregnancy will vary depending on your individual needs, your safety, and the experience of your health care professional.

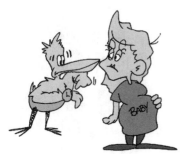

My A1C is 6.8% on 2 shots of insulin a day. My diabetes team is recommending 3 to 4 injections a day now that I am pregnant. Why?

▼
TIP:

First of all, congratulations on your efforts to control your blood glucose! A 6.8% A1C level is very good. It is important to note, though, that the goals for diabetes control are different when you are pregnant. When you're pregnant you want the lowest A1C possible, without putting yourself at an excessive risk for hypoglycemia. Normal A1C is usually considered below 6%, though individual lab analysis may vary. Your diabetes team is probably recommending 3–4 injections daily to help you fine-tune your insulin regimen. This might be to help you control your after-meal blood glucose a little better, or it might be to lower your risk of hypoglycemia, or it might be both. Self blood glucose monitoring (up to 8 times daily) is recommended to continuously evaluate your diabetes care plan and assist with any necessary changes in a prompt manner.

*M*y endocrinologist is recommending an insulin pump to help me control my diabetes while I am pregnant. How will it help?

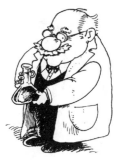

▼
TIP:

B y providing very tight blood glucose control. An insulin pump is a mechanical device attached to tubing and an infusion set that infuses insulin directly under your skin. The pump sends insulin through the tubing/catheter at a preprogrammed, continuous (basal) rate, as well as in larger insulin amounts (bolus) programmed by the user to cover any carbohydrate intake from snacks or meals. Many health care professionals recommend the use of insulin pumps during pregnancy because they feel that pump therapy closely mimics the insulin release of a normal pancreas. Ideally, you would start pump therapy *before* pregnancy to achieve good glucose control before you conceive.

Insulin pump therapy has been used safely in both type 1 and type 2 diabetes. The ability to adjust and deliver insulin in increments smaller than 1.0 unit makes it easier to fine-tune insulin delivery during very insulin-sensitive periods (such as the 1st trimester, especially in type 1 diabetes), as well as in insulin-resistant states, which occurs in type 2, gestational diabetes (GDM), and during the 2nd and 3rd trimesters in type 1 diabetes. You will want to evaluate the expense of insulin pump therapy and determine your health care coverage for the device and supplies. The expense may not be as feasible if you have gestational diabetes, since GDM usually disappears once the baby is delivered, making insulin pump therapy a short-term investment.

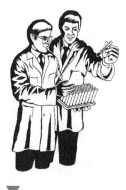

I don't have type 1 diabetes, but my doctor says I will need insulin during my pregnancy. Why?

▼
TIP:

Because insulin is the best and safest way to control your blood glucose while you're pregnant. Many women have successfully used nutrition, exercise, and diabetes pills to manage type 2 diabetes. However, oral diabetes medications are usually not used during pregnancy because of the possible risk of complications. More research is needed to determine whether or not diabetes pills are safe for women who are pregnant. Insulin, on the other hand, has been safely used to manage diabetes in pregnancy for years.

Ideally, you should start an intensive insulin regimen (3–4 injections daily) or perhaps insulin pump therapy *before* you are pregnant to get your blood glucose under control. Keep in mind that insulin resistance increases in type 2 diabetes during pregnancy, as well as in type 1 and gestational diabetes in the 2nd and 3rd trimesters. This is a result of weight gain and contrainsulin hormones produced by the placenta. Remember to increase your self-blood glucose checks up to 8 times a day to keep yourself and your diabetes care team aware of where you are in your control.

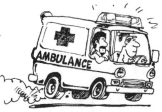

O nce I became pregnant I started intensive insulin therapy. My doctor told me I needed to have a medication called glucagon *available just in case I needed it. What is glucagon?*

▼
TIP:

Glucagon is a hormone injection used as an emergency treatment for hypoglycemia (low blood sugar). During pregnancy, you run a higher risk of hypoglycemia due to lower blood sugar goals, lower sensitivity to the symptoms of hypoglycemia (hypoglycemia unawareness), and the use of your glucose stores by the fetus. Glucagon is used when you have severe hypoglycemia in which you are unable to swallow, perhaps confused, or have passed out due to hypoglycemia. It works by causing the liver to make glucose and usually takes effect within 15 minutes. Once you are alert and able to eat, monitor your blood glucose levels carefully and eat a car-bohydrate snack, such as crackers. Keep in mind that a full syringe of glucagon will be too much for anyone weighing less than 120 pounds. In this case, it's best to give 1/2 of the shot and then wait 15 minutes before giving the rest.

A glucagon kit is recommended for anyone with type 1 diabetes, regardless of whether or not you are pregnant. If you have type 2 or gestational diabetes, your diabetes care team should assess whether or not you need glucagon. A prescription is required to obtain glucagon at the pharmacy and your physician may want to write the prescrip-tion for a "Glucagon Emergency Kit" that contains a syringe and is ready to be mixed and injected. Since you will be in no shape to give yourself glucagon when you need it, your family members or signifi-cant others will need to be fully educated on how to give you a glucagon injection and know the location of the kit, which is usually refrigerated.

Chapter 5
BABY STEPS
Physical Activity During Pregnancy

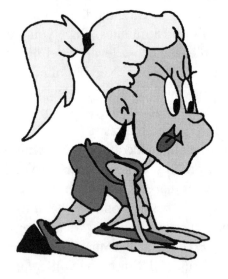

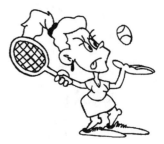

*S*hould I exercise while I'm pregnant?

▼
TIP:

Yes. The American College of Obstetricians and Gynecologists recommends 30 minutes or more of moderate exercise a day on most, if not all, days of the week for pregnant women who don't have medical or obstetric complications (see page 48 for a list of complications that would keep you from exercising). If your physician has evaluated you and finds that your diabetes is well controlled without complications, physical activity can provide a variety of benefits in terms of both your pregnancy and your diabetes.

Moderate exercise helps you prepare for the physical demands of labor and childbirth. Exercise can help improve your muscle tone, circulation, and heart function, as well as provide you with a feeling of mental and physical well-being. Women who are physically fit find that their recovery after childbirth is faster and easier. Exercise also helps increase the efficiency of your body's own insulin, meaning that if you do require insulin during pregnancy, exercise may allow you to use a smaller dose.

Discuss a program of physical activity during pregnancy with your physician and diabetes team. They can notify you of any special limitations or considerations, as well as provide you with specific guidelines for taking care of your diabetes as you exercise.

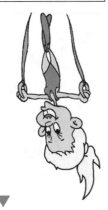

A *re there any pregnancy-related*
complications that would prevent me
from exercising?

▼
TIP:

Y es. Exercising with some complications could put you and your child at undue risk. Such complications include:

- significant heart or lung disease
- being at risk for premature labor
- experiencing premature labor during your current pregnancy
- multiple gestation (twins or more) at risk for premature labor
- persistent 2nd- or 3rd-trimester bleeding
- placenta previa (a condition where the placenta would precede the baby's exit from the womb after 26 weeks into the pregnancy)
- ruptured membranes
- incompetent cervix
- preeclampsia/pregnancy-induced hypertension (high blood pressure)

Having any of these conditions is an indication that you should not participate in aerobic exercise while you're pregnant. If you have been diagnosed with any of the above, or feel that you may be at risk, talk with your diabetes health care team about the precautions you should take.

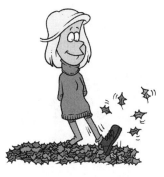

I wasn't physically active before my pregnancy. What is the best exercise for a diabetic pregnancy?

▼
TIP:

B ecause you were relatively inactive before your pregnancy, it is wise to have your obstetrician evaluate you and make recommendations for specific types of physical activity during your pregnancy. Physical activity provides many pregnancy health benefits and assists in blood glucose control. Walking is considered one of the best forms of physical activity for pregnant women. Brisk walking will provide you with a good total body workout and should be relatively easy on your joints and muscles. Swimming, water aerobics, and prenatal stretching classes offer other opportunities for you to gradually begin a program of physical activity. Arm exercises might be another option. If you have your physician's OK, your goal should be to accumulate 30 minutes or more of moderate exercise on most, if not all, days of the week. Be sure to check your blood glucose before, during, and after your exercise session and make adjustments in your meal plan if needed.

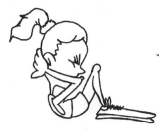

*W*hich exercises should I avoid now that I'm pregnant?

▼
TIP:

Anything that puts your body under unnecessary stress. Pregnancy means many changes in your body, which means changes in your ability to exercise. Pregnancy hormones cause the ligaments that support your joints to become relaxed, so you should avoid jerky, bouncy, or high-impact motions. Because you are carrying extra pounds (most of them in the front of your body), your center of gravity has shifted. This may place stress on the joints and muscles in your pelvis and lower back. In addition, those extra pregnancy pounds will mean that your body has to work harder during exercise than before. Don't overdo it!

Although you and your physician should go over your plans for physical activity, in general, it is best to avoid activities with a high risk of falling (gymnastics, horseback riding, downhill skiing, tennis, racquet-ball, etc.), those with a high risk of injury to your abdomen (ice hockey, soccer, and basketball), and, if you're not used to exercise, exercises that put stress on your lower body (bicycling, strength straining with your legs, etc.). In addition, you should avoid scuba diving because the fetus is at increased risk for decompression sickness during this activity.

Certain forms of exercise may involve uncomfortable positions and movements that may be harmful for pregnant women. For example, after the 1st trimester, the expanding uterus may affect circulation to the fetus, so it's best to avoid exercises that require you to lie flat on your back.

Although physical activity is good for both your pregnancy and your diabetes, be careful and choose the best form of exercise for your health and that of your baby.

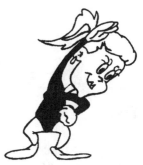

When is the best time for me to exercise?

▼
TIP:

This depends on your diabetes. In most cases, exercise lowers blood glucose by helping your body's cells become more sensitive to insulin. It may be best to take part in physical activity directly after a meal when your blood glucose level will be at its highest. Women with gestational diabetes may find that taking a walk after breakfast is especially helpful in controlling their morning rise in blood glucose. If you are taking insulin, you should avoid vigorous physical activity at the time your insulin is reaching its peak. Remember that exercise can have a blood glucose lowering effect for up to 24 hours after you've stopped exercising, so continue to check your blood glucose frequently.

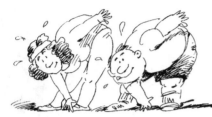

*H*ow do I avoid low blood sugar while I'm exercising?

TIP:

Don't take any chances. Being pregnant can make you more prone to low blood glucose (hypoglycemia), and you may experience hypoglycemia if you delay a meal, skip a snack or meal, or exercise more than usual. To prevent hypoglycemia, check your blood glucose frequently—before, during, and after physical activity if necessary.

- **Before you exercise**—Check your blood glucose. If it is over 240 mg/dl and you take insulin, follow up by checking your urine for ketones. If ketones are present, this means you do not have enough insulin in your system. You may need more insulin, so contact your health care team and do not exercise until your ketone levels have returned to trace or negative amounts.

  If your blood glucose is less than 100 mg/dl before you begin a 30-minute session of physical activity, eat a small snack with 15 grams of carbohydrate such as 1 small muffin, 1 small piece of fruit, or 1/2 an English muffin.

- **While you are exercising**—Be alert for the signs of hypo- glycemia, such as headache, shakiness, confusion, sweatiness, irritability, fatigue, hunger, and personality change. Check your blood glucose. If it is below 70 mg/dl, treat it with 10–15 grams of carbohydrate. Good sources are glucose tablets or gel, 4 ounces of fruit juice or regular soft drink, 6–8 ounces of fat-free or low- fat milk, or 5–7 Lifesavers. Recheck your blood glucose within 15 minutes and treat again if necessary. Do not resume exercising until your blood glucose is back to at least 100 mg/dl.

- **After you exercise**—Physical activity continues to have a blood glucose lowering effect up to 24 hours after you've exercised. Continue to monitor your blood glucose on a regular schedule and be alert for the signs and symptoms of hypoglycemia.

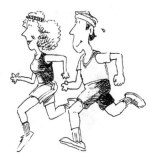

I *have type 1 diabetes and routinely jog 6 miles a day. I just found out that I am pregnant. Can I continue my daily jog?*

▼
TIP:

Physical activity is highly recommended for pregnant women with diabetes, particularly if you have been in good shape before becoming pregnant. Check with your physician for a complete evaluation as soon as possible. If your diabetes is under control, without complications, it is likely you'll be able to continue your routine, as long as it is comfortable and safe for you and the baby. At some point, you may need to switch to a more low-impact form of exercise, such as brisk walking. If you have a history or risk of preterm labor or fetal growth restriction, your obstetrician may advise you to reduce your activity in the 2nd and 3rd trimesters.

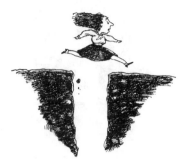

I would like to continue exercising while I'm pregnant, as long as it's safe. What are some warning signs that I should stop exercising?

▼
TIP:

B e alert for the following warning signs that you should stop exercising while you're pregnant:

- Signs and symptoms of hypoglycemia (low blood sugar)
- Vaginal bleeding
- Shortness of breath before you exercise
- Dizziness
- Headache
- Chest pain
- Muscle weakness
- Calf pain or swelling
- Preterm labor
- Decreased movement of the fetus
- Amniotic fluid leakage
- Uterine cramping without bleeding

If you do experience any of these symptoms, stop exercising and contact your health care team.

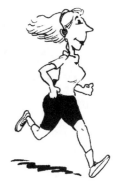

I was just told I have gestational diabetes. The diabetes educator told me that exercise would help control my blood glucose levels. How?

▼
TIP:

Physical activity lowers blood glucose by helping the body cells become more sensitive to insulin, which helps control your blood glucose. Gestational diabetes (GDM) is a form of diabetes that appears during pregnancy and usually disappears after the baby is born. Its exact cause is unknown, but it may be related to pregnancy hormones that block insulin's action in the mother's body, causing insulin resistance. If insulin is not working efficiently, glucose builds up in the blood. This can potentially cause complications in the baby, such as large birth weight, low blood sugar, breathing difficulties at birth, and jaundice. Treatment for gestational diabetes is geared toward keeping blood glucose levels as close to normal as possible and involves a healthy eating plan, physical activity, and insulin, if necessary.

Taking a brisk walk for 20–30 minutes after meals can be a big help in controlling blood glucose, particularly since glucose levels are highest after meals. Pregnancy hormones are often at higher levels in the morning, making women with gestational diabetes more prone to higher blood glucose values in the morning. In this situation, a brisk walk after breakfast can be very helpful in keeping blood glucose levels in control.

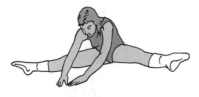

*W*hat should be included in a good exercise routine for a pregnant woman with diabetes?

▼
TIP:

Lots of things. Pregnant women with diabetes reap many benefits from exercise, such as improved muscle tone, circulation, and heart function, as well as a feeling of mental and physical well-being. Exercise also helps your body use its own insulin more efficiently, meaning that if you do require insulin during pregnancy, exercise may allow you to use a smaller dose. If you have been evaluated by your physician and have been given the OK to include more physical activity in your daily routine, be sure to consider the following points:

- Check your blood glucose levels before, during, and after an exercise session.
- Always have a fast-acting form of carbohydrate and/or a snack available to treat low blood sugar.
- If it's been some time since you've exercised, start slowly and work up to the recommended goal of 30 minutes a day of moderate exercise, such as brisk walking or light arm exercises.
- Drink plenty of water before, during, and after an exercise session.
- Always begin each exercise session with a warm-up period that includes such activities as careful stretching.
- Don't go overboard. As a general rule, your pulse should not go over 140 beats per minute during your exercise session.
- After you exercise, allow enough time to cool down and reduce your activity level gradually.

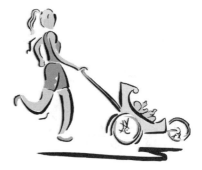

*H*ow can I become more
physically fit after the
baby is born?

▼
TIP:

B y resuming the activity schedule you had before you were pregnant. Just remember to take it slowly. Many of the changes
your body experiences during pregnancy persist from 4–6 weeks
after you have your baby. Plus, your body will require time to
recover from the hard work involved in labor and delivery.

Because physical activity is so beneficial to your general health
and diabetes control, it is very important to resume an exercise routine after you check with your physician. Although recovery may be
a bit longer after a cesarean delivery, your prepregnancy exercise
routines should be resumed gradually as soon as it is physically and
medically safe. A quick return to physical activity after childbirth
will help you get your body back into shape and has been linked to
a reduced risk of postpartum depression.

If you have had gestational diabetes during your pregnancy, it is
important for you to realize that you are at high risk for developing
type 2 diabetes later in life. For this reason, you should continue to
follow a healthy meal plan and lose any excess weight you may
have gained. Physical activity is especially beneficial for you
because exercise helps your body use glucose more effectively,
and this reduces your risk for developing type 2 diabetes.

Chapter 6
A CLOSE CHECK ON
DIABETES CONTROL

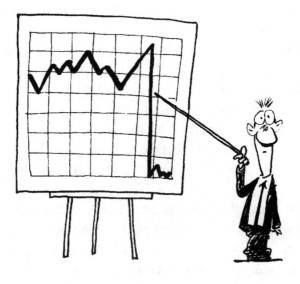

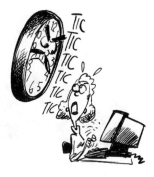

I had diabetes before I was pregnant.
Now that I am pregnant, how often
should I monitor my blood glucose?

▼
TIP:

Most health care professionals recommend that a woman with preexisting diabetes (both type 1 and type 2) who becomes pregnant monitor her blood glucose levels up to 8 times daily. In terms of your day-to-day routine, you should probably monitor:

■ before each meal
■ 1 or 2 hours after each meal
■ at bedtime
■ occasionally at 2–3 A.M.

Monitoring your blood glucose frequently gives you detailed information about your blood glucose control, helps you identify changes in your control (such as hypoglycemia or hyperglycemia), gives you information about the effects of meals and other events (such as exercise) on your blood glucose, and provides you with feedback for changes in your insulin therapy.

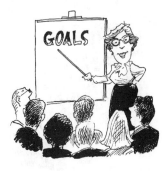

*W*hat are the blood glucose goals
for women who are pregnant?

▼
TIP:

W hen women who do not have diabetes are pregnant, their
blood glucose levels tend to be lower than non-pregnant
levels. It follows that when a woman who has diabetes gets pregnant, she'll aim for lower glucose levels as well. The following table
gives the recommendations for diabetes and pregnancy blood glucose goals from the American Diabetes Association. Whole blood
values reflect a blood sample that is taken and measured by a meter
using a whole blood sample. A plasma value would be a serum-
blood sample for glucose taken by a laboratory (or a fingerstick
value using a meter that converts the whole blood reading to a
plasma-correlated value). Plasma values usually read approximately
10–15% higher than whole blood values.

Blood Glucose Goals for Diabetes and Pregnancy		
Timing	**Whole Blood Value**	**Plasma Value**
Fasting	60–90mg/dl	69–104mg/dl
Before meals	60–105mg/dl	69–121mg/dl
1 hours after meals	100–120mg/dl	115–138mg/dl
2 AM–6 AM	60–120mg/dl	69–138mg/dl

Adapted from *Medical Management of Pregnancy Complicated by Diabetes*, 3rd ed.,
ADA, 2000.

Discuss appropriate blood glucose goals with your health care team.

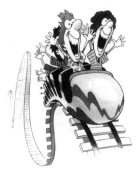

*W*hat should my A1C (Hemoglobin A1C) be while I am pregnant?

▼
TIP:

An A1C (Hemoglobin A1C) is a blood test that can predict average blood glucose levels for about 8–12 weeks. People without diabetes generally have an A1C of less than 6%, though this usually drops to less than 5% during pregnancy. Women with diabetes should strive for "near normal" A1C's prior to, as well as during, pregnancy. Studies show that if you can keep your A1C to 1% above normal or lower, the risk of birth defects is about the same as for someone without diabetes. Keep in mind that the rates of each complication continue to decrease the lower A1C test levels go. It is essential for you and your diabetes care team to establish the lowest possible A1C goal for you, without putting you at excessive risk for hypoglycemia. Fine-tuning all areas of your diabetes treatment plan will be helpful in achieving this goal.

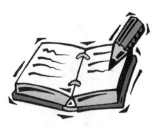

I have gestational diabetes and I'm monitoring my blood sugars 2 hours after each meal. Why is that important?

▼
TIP:

Since you didn't have diabetes before you were pregnant, it is helpful to see how eating affects your blood glucose control. It is essential for you to partner with a registered dietitian (RD) to develop a meal plan that is right for you. Even if you closely follow the meal plan, normal pregnancy hormones, as well as the weight you're bound to gain while pregnant, will cause your blood glucose levels to fluctuate. *Do not* stop eating or skip meals to control your blood glucose. Insulin therapy may be necessary to control your glucose levels. See page 41 for guidelines on beginning insulin therapy with GDM.

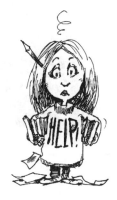

My doctor wants me to report blood glucose results on a weekly basis. Is this really necessary?

▼
TIP:

Yes! Most health care teams like to study blood glucose results on a 1–2 week basis during pregnancy. Depending on how often you have appointments, the physician who is managing your diabetes may have you call, fax, or email in your blood glucose numbers if you are not seeing him/her during a particular week. If you have 2 blood glucose numbers in a 1-week period that are higher than the recommended goals, quick adjustments to your treatment plan need to be made. For women with gestational diabetes (GDM), blood glucose numbers that do not meet goals may indicate you need to start taking insulin. For women with type 1, type 2, and GDM who take insulin, adjustments are typically needed at least every 2 weeks, although this may vary from person to person. Because of the effects of contrainsulin hormones, as well as other factors that "aggravate" blood glucose levels, close monitoring and frequent adjustments to your treatment plan will probably be necessary throughout your pregnancy.

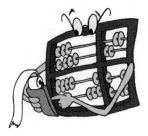

I have gestational diabetes and have been monitoring my blood sugar levels for about 4 weeks. All of my readings have been within recommended goals. Do I need to keep checking?

▼
TIP:

Yes. Your good glucose control is good for both you and the baby. As your pregnancy moves along, your need for insulin will increase. This is due, in part, to a continuing increase in the hormones produced by your placenta and various other maternal hormones. As these hormones and the weight in your abdomen increase, so does the need for insulin. Women with preexisting diabetes will need double or sometimes even triple the insulin they did before they were pregnant. You will need to monitor your blood sugar levels to be sure that your body can cope with these increasing demands for insulin. If your blood glucose starts to rise, it allows you and your diabetes team to immediately modify your treatment plan as necessary to keep you and your baby healthy!

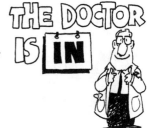

I am pregnant and have gestational diabetes. After lunch my blood glucose was 145 mg/dl. My friend with diabetes says that blood glucose level is OK, but my doctor says it isn't. Who's right?

▼
TIP:

In a way, both your friend and your doctor are right—depending on the situation. When it comes to goals for pregnant women with diabetes, your doctor has the right answer. Your reading of 135 mg/dl is higher than the recommended pregnancy goal. See page 60 for the American Diabetes Association's blood glucose goals for pregnancy.

Your friend, on the other hand, may be thinking about the *recommended* goals for glucose control, without regard to pregnancy. The normal goals for people with diabetes who are not pregnant are slightly higher than pregnancy goals. Discuss any concerns you have with your health care team. When your glucose levels are outside the recommended range for pregnancy and diabetes, your treatment plan should probably be adjusted.

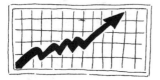

*M*y A1C was 9.0% when I got
pregnant. Will my baby be OK?

▼
TIP:

This depends on what you're doing about it now. A number of studies have shown that a high A1C level in early pregnancy can lead to a 2–5 times higher risk of birth defects and miscarriages. Generally, the higher the A1C, the greater the risk for these complications. It's recommended that you get your blood glucose under control *before* you are pregnant. In fact, normalizing blood glucose levels before and during pregnancy reduces your risk of pregnancy-related complications to that of the nondiabetic population. Now that you are pregnant, it is absolutely necessary that your blood glucose be controlled. Ideally, you should work with a team of health care professionals to help you manage your diabetes during pregnancy. This team should include:

■ your primary care physician or endocrinologist
■ an obstetrician
■ a nurse educator (preferably a certified diabetes educator, or CDE)
■ a social worker
■ a registered dietitian
■ a pediatrician or neonatologist

There are a variety of tests designed to check for birth defects, including ultrasonography and amniocentesis. If you plan to become pregnant again in the future, work with your health care team and have your blood glucose under control *before* pregnancy!

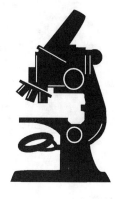

I have gestational diabetes, I'm 36 weeks pregnant, and I'm using insulin. My doctor just did a fructosamine test to monitor my blood glucose control. What does this mean?

▼
TIP:

A *fructosamine* test shows the amount of glucose attached to your protein molecules, which is a good indicator of your continuous glucose levels over a 2-week period. Some health care professionals use the results of this test to monitor short-term changes in glucose control, mostly to see how well adjustments to your plan are going. When it comes to pregnancy and diabetes, you want to achieve good control as quick as you can. A fructosamine test is a good way to get reliable, continuous blood glucose readings over a relatively short period of time.

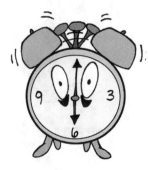

*M*y *diabetes team recommends urine ketone testing every morning. Is this necessary?*

▼
TIP:

Yes. Ketones appear when your body can't break down the glucose in your bloodstream *or* if there is not enough glucose available to meet your energy needs. When this happens, your body begins to use stored fat for energy, which results in ketones (acid substances) in your bloodstream. Ketone testing each morning can help you detect a condition called "starvation ketones," which means there is not enough glucose in your bloodstream for you and the fetus. If the condition persists over a few days, your diabetes health care team may recommend an increase in calories, perhaps with your bedtime snack. A condition called "ketoacidosis" can occur if ketones get built up in your bloodstream. Prompt troubleshooting of high blood glucose levels is essential while you are pregnant, since ketoacidosis can occur very quickly and at lower blood glucose levels than normal. Regular ketone testing done each morning, as well as when you have high blood glucose, can help prevent a serious medical situation.

I have type 2 diabetes and have been using my forearm for blood glucose checks. I just found out I am pregnant and my doctor recommended fingerstick glucose checks instead. Why?

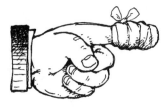

▼
TIP:

B ecause the fingerstick method is more accurate. Your blood glucose readings change during the course of the day, due to things such as food, medication, illness, stress, and exercise. Glucose circulates through your body in the bloodstream, first through your arteries, then to the capillaries (such as in your fingers), and finally your veins. The blood in your arteries has the highest glucose levels, followed by capillary blood, and then the blood in your veins. Blood also flows faster in your fingers than it does in alternative sites, such as your thigh, calf, forearm, upper arm, or hand. So what does this mean? It means that alternative site glucose values can lag behind fingerstick glucose values; changes are seen sooner in a fingerstick sample. When your blood glucose rises after a meal, or you suffer a sudden onset of hypoglycemia, you'll notice more quickly by using fingerstick samples. This is especially important when you're pregnant, since the recommended goals for glucose control are "tighter" than normal. This includes glucose values both before and after eating (see page 60 for diabetes/pregnancy glucose goals). In addition, hypoglycemia is often more frequent and more severe during pregnancy. Because of this, your doctor may prefer you use the fingerstick method to get the fastest, most reliable reading possible.

Chapter 7
PREGNANCY
PEACE OF MIND

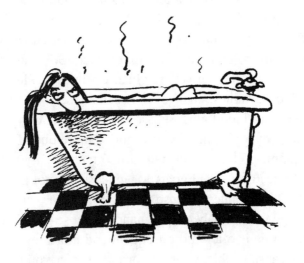

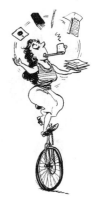

I have always had excellent control of my
diabetes, but this pregnancy has turned
my life—and diabetes management—upside
down. What can I do to get back in control?

▼
TIP:

That depends. Diabetes is a complex condition and the physical
and hormonal changes of pregnancy can provide even more
challenges to your management plan. It's important to accept the
fact that your diabetes may not always respond the way you'd like,
even though you are doing everything "by the book." You may find
yourself feeling especially anxious when your diabetes control is
less than perfect during your pregnancy, or if you have to begin taking insulin or increase your previous insulin dosage. Rest assured
that your diabetes has not gotten worse; actually, your blood glucose
is responding as expected to the contrainsulin hormones released by
your growing placenta.

To preserve your sense of well-being and control, be sure to stay
actively involved in your medical care. Ask your health care team
questions when needed and communicate your concerns clearly.
Realize that your body will respond differently now that you're
pregnant and pat yourself on the back every day for your hard work
and your efforts to give birth to a healthy baby!

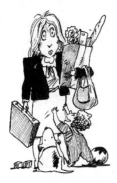

Trying to take care of a two-year-old and keep my diabetes under control while I'm pregnant seems impossible. Is it?

▼
TIP:

Raising a small child while you are pregnant is very demanding—to say nothing of the added challenge of keeping your diabetes under control. It's understandable that you may feel overwhelmed at times. Rather than trying to manage everything yourself, this is the time to practice what mental health professionals call "positive selfishness." Accept offers of help from others whenever they're made. If your child's friend invites him over for a play date, accept happily and use the time to relax and regroup. Don't be reluctant to ask others for help. Perhaps your mother can help by cooking a meal every once in a while, or your husband can help more often with the household chores and shopping. If you can't afford to hire a babysitter, try trading childcare duties with a neighbor or friend. This will free up some time for you to enjoy a nap or a break at the movies. If you take care of yourself first, you'll be more likely to have energy left to take care of the other important things in your life, including your diabetes.

I'm constantly worried about how my blood glucose is affecting the baby. What can I do to relieve this?

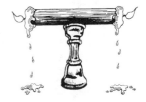

▼
TIP:

K eep in mind that pregnancy is a time of apprehension—and excitement—for women, whether they have diabetes or not. As a woman with diabetes, all the decisions you make regarding your health and diabetes care have an impact on the health of your baby as well. It's no surprise that your anxiety level is high! Remember that advances in diabetes and neonatal care mean that the odds are greatly in your favor for having a healthy baby, as long as you work to keep your blood glucose levels as near normal as possible during your pregnancy. An out of range blood glucose reading every once in a while isn't likely to be a disaster. Checking your blood glucose levels often will help you make the necessary adjustments in your management plan.

Share your anxiety over your baby's health with your medical team. The frequent medical tests you undergo during your pregnancy (ultrasounds, fetal stress tests, etc.) can go a long way toward reassuring you that your baby is developing as he or she should. If you find that your worries are just too much to handle, it may be helpful to seek professional help so you'll be better able to cope with the stress—and joy—of pregnancy.

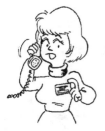

I would love to talk with another woman who has managed a pregnancy with diabetes. How can I get in touch with someone to share experiences?

▼
TIP:

Talking with other women who have experienced pregnancy with diabetes can help you gain perspective and valuable information, as well as peace of mind. Often, just talking about concerns, ranging from the challenges of frequent blood glucose monitoring to the misery of morning sickness, can reassure you that things are going as they should. Internet chat rooms are one way to get in touch with others in your situation. Support groups can also provide lots of practical advice. Check with your physician, midwife, or diabetes care team. While they probably won't be able to share actual patient names and phone numbers with you because of privacy issues, they will be able to point you in the right direction. It may be as simple as taking the initiative to post a sign in the office of your obstetrician. You may also want to contact the maternity service of the hospital in which you plan to deliver for information on their support groups. If you enjoy sharing your experiences with other women, think about helping others after you deliver your baby by coming back and sharing your success!

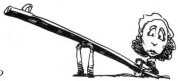

My husband doesn't seem to understand why I need to check my blood glucose so often and watch what I eat so carefully. Is this typical?

▼
TIP:

Yes, it is. As you know, proper diabetes care during pregnancy takes a lot of time, thought, and extra effort—something that even the most loving of husbands may find difficult to understand. Often times, soon-to-be fathers feel "left out" of the details surrounding their wife's pregnancy. Your husband may also be feeling anxious about your health and the health of the baby. And let's not forget that a new baby can bring immense changes to your finances and your personal relationship—additional sources of anxiety.

Ask your husband to join you at as many of your health care appointments as possible. This will give him an opportunity to learn more about what's required for a healthy pregnancy with diabetes and a chance to let him feel like he's a bigger part of your support team.

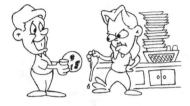

Will the stress I'm experiencing with this pregnancy affect my blood glucose?

▼
TIP:

Yes. The increased demands of diabetes, as well as the natural anxiety and anticipation that come with pregnancy, can affect your blood glucose. Stress, whether it's mental or physical, can cause your body to release hormones that work against insulin. As a result, your blood glucose will rise. On the other hand, you may also find that your stress is keeping you from eating as well as you should, which can lead to low blood glucose levels. If the extra stress you're feeling during pregnancy is affecting your blood glucose, go back to the basics of good diabetes management—proper nutrition, physical activity, and plenty of rest. Relaxation techniques, such as deep breathing and meditation, can also improve your mental outlook *and* your blood glucose levels.

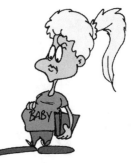

Sometimes I have very negative feelings about this pregnancy, mostly because of the extra demands it makes on my diabetes care routine. What can I do to improve my attitude?

▼

TIP:

First, you need to realize that what you are feeling is normal. All pregnant women, whether they have diabetes or not, experience both strong negative and positive feelings. Many things cause emotional swings during pregnancy, not just the extra demands on your diabetes care. Pregnancy hormones play a big part in your irritability, mood swings, weepiness, and misgivings about having a baby. On the other hand, at times you may find yourself feeling calm, happy, and excited about your future new arrival.

As with any stressful situation, it helps to talk about it—either with your significant other, a close friend, or a member of your health care team. If you are feeling overwhelmed by the demands of pregnancy, ask for help at home or work. Be sure to get enough rest and eat well. Physical activity can also relieve stress. A mini "getaway," such as a long walk, movie, or good book can help when you need a break.

If you feel that your negative feelings are overwhelming you, don't be reluctant to seek some professional counseling. Your anxiety about your health care routine is understandable. Working through your negative feelings will help you take good care of yourself and your baby.

Chapter 8
NINE-MONTH
SURVEILLANCE

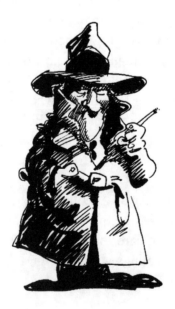

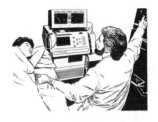

I have gestational diabetes and am due to deliver in about 2 weeks. My doctor says I need an ultrasound. Why now?

▼
TIP:

Because the results can help your doctor plan for your delivery. Ultrasonography uses sound to create an image of the fetus, which can then be used to check for problems. It also helps determine how your baby is growing and how much it weighs. If you have diabetes, you run a higher risk of delivering a macrosomic (large) infant. On the other hand, if you had preexisting diabetes and any blood pressure or general heart problems, there's a chance that fetal growth might actually be lower than normal. An ultrasound can determine whether or not your physician will need to take extra steps during delivery. Although ultrasound estimates can be off by about 10%, it can still be useful to predict size and potentially difficult deliveries.

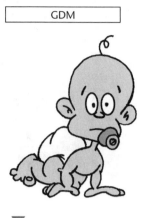

I was just diagnosed with gestational diabetes and my doctor says my baby is "big." Is it too late to do anything about it?

TIP:

Not at all—but you need to get things in gear right away! Although you will not be able to decrease the size of your baby, there are ways you can slow its faster-than-average growth to more normal rates. Your first goal should be getting your blood glucose under control (see page 60 for recommended goals during pregnancy). Good blood glucose control is essential. More than likely, it is hyperglycemia (high blood glucose levels) that has led to your baby's large size. It is important to understand what causes high blood glucose during pregnancy, including:

- Physical stress, including the stress caused by maternal hormones
- Carbohydrate intake
- Abdominal weight, which will increase during pregnancy

These are normal, essential components of your pregnancy. Work with your health care team on a plan that will help you keep your blood glucose levels under control. Talk with a diabetes educator to build a plan for healthy eating, physical activity, and blood glucose and urine-ketone monitoring schedules. A registered dietitian can help you with healthy meal planning, which is absolutely essential for women with GDM. Most important, stay focused and diligent, and everything else will fall in line.

I *have kidney disease related to my*
diabetes. Will this affect my pregnancy?

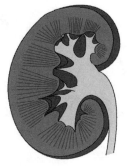

▼
TIP:

It may. What may be more important is how your pregnancy will affect your kidney condition. Women with nephropathy (kidney disease) who are pregnant run a higher risk of hypertension (high blood pressure) and problems with edema (fluid retention), which can require serious medical attention and lead to toxemia. You should be evaluated before you are pregnant to determine the risks involved with your particular case. The degree of your kidney disease should be considered and the risks of pregnancy should be discussed. If your proteinuria (protein in the urine) is greater than 2 grams per 24 hours, you probably should not become pregnant. If you do become pregnant, careful education and follow-up are essential and necessary for the best possible outcome.

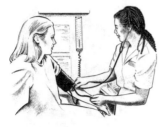

I have a history of high blood pressure and I'm 6 weeks pregnant. Will the pregnancy affect my blood pressure?

▼
TIP:

More than likely, yes. In fact, it is best to have an evaluation before you are pregnant. A number of medications for high blood pressure are not safe for use while you are pregnant. Some may even lead to birth defects. As your pregnancy progresses, you should monitor your blood pressure very closely. Poorly controlled blood pressure can restrict the growth of your baby by lowering circulation across the placenta. Poorly controlled blood pressure may also lead to toxemia, which is high blood pressure with protein in the urine and swelling from fluid retention. Work closely with your health care team to monitor your blood pressure status.

*M*y doctor says an alpha-feto protein test is recommended for all women with diabetes during pregnancy. Why?

▼
TIP:

An alpha-feto protein (AFP) test is given to women with pre-existing diabetes as a way to screen for any birth defects. High levels of alpha-feto protein in your bloodstream can be the sign of an "open" fetal defect (such as spina bifida) that is usually linked to poor blood glucose control in the early weeks of pregnancy. High alpha-feto protein can also indicate that there is more than one fetus present, a miscarriage is likely, or the fetus has died. Low levels of alpha-feto protein may indicate a chromosome-related problem, such as Down's syndrome. Generally, chromosome problems are not related to glucose control. If you do have an AFP test, it is important you do it between 16 and 18 weeks for the best possible accuracy. Keep in mind that just because the AFP test gives high or low readings, it does not always mean there is a problem—it just means you need more testing.

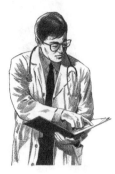

My doctor says I will be having non-stress tests every week after I get to 32 weeks of pregnancy. Is this necessary?

▼

TIP:

A nonstress test, or NST, is used as a way to see how your fetus is doing in the uterus. Basically, the test monitors the heart rate of the fetus after it moves. If the heart rate goes up after movement, this is considered a "reactive" NST and it is a good sign everything is all right. If the heart rate does not go up, it is considered "nonreactive," which may suggest there is a problem. If the fetus does not move at all, your doctor will want to do more testing. Try to remember that if the fetus doesn't move and you get a "nonreactive" reading, the fetus may just be sleeping. If you're healthy, your doctor may suggest NSTs after 35 weeks. If you have heart disease and/or hypertension, your doctor may want to run NSTs as early as 28 weeks.

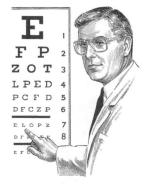

I had diabetes before my pregnancy and have read that I need to visit my ophthalmologist 3 times during my pregnancy. Why?

▼
TIP:

First of all, you do need to visit the ophthalmologist while you're pregnant. How many times is up to your ophthalmologist. These visits are necessary to detect any changes in your retina and provide treatment before the changes cause permanent vision damage. If you have pre-existing diabetes, you should have a baseline eye examination by a retinal specialist (ophthalmologist) during the 1st trimester of your pregnancy. This eye exam should be complete, with dilated pupils and visualization of the retinal circulation to determine the health of your eyes. Further exams during your pregnancy can help keep track of how the pregnancy is affecting your eyes. Your ophthalmologist will recommend more follow-up eye exams as necessary. Ideally, you should have an eye examination before you are pregnant, so that if there are any problems, they can be controlled before you are pregnant.

Chapter 9
LABOR DAY

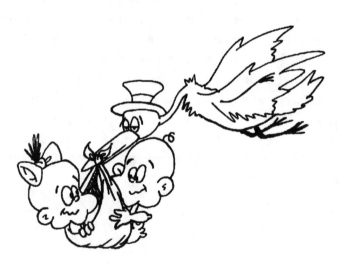

How will labor and delivery affect my blood glucose control?

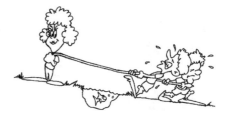

▼
TIP:

In a variety of ways, and not just for you, but for the baby as well. If your blood glucose is high during labor, this excess glucose can cross the placenta to your baby. Your baby will react by stimulating his or her own pancreatic insulin. After delivery, this extra insulin can cause low blood sugars since the baby has been removed from your supply of glucose.

Your blood glucose levels will also depend on what type of delivery you have. If you have a cesarean section, your blood glucose may rise from the stress on your body caused by surgery. On the other hand, if you deliver vaginally, your glucose levels will drop since the delivery will have the same effect as exercise. In fact, once labor starts, your insulin requirements will temporarily disappear and your glucose needs will remain pretty constant. Many women with gestational diabetes do not need insulin during labor and delivery. Your blood sugar should be checked every hour while you're in labor to ensure things are under control.

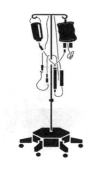

My *y doctor mentioned I might be put on an insulin drip while I'm in labor. Is this necessary?*

▼
TIP:

This depends on you and your situation. If you are using a pump, then your medical team will probably want you to continue using the pump, with some adjustments. If you are not using a pump, however, an insulin drip will be a good idea. Keep in mind that your need for insulin will drop once you go into labor. If you've been injecting insulin during your pregnancy, these injections can't give you the very tight control an insulin drip can provide. By infusing insulin (as well as saline solution and glucose) directly into your veins in precise increments, your medical team can tightly control your blood glucose levels during labor and delivery. You and your medical team will need to frequently monitor your glucose levels to decide what adjustments need to be made. If you have gestational diabetes (GDM), you probably will not need an insulin drip, but you will still need to frequently monitor your blood glucose levels. No matter what type of diabetes you have, your insulin needs will drop drastically after delivery, so any insulin infusions will need to be stopped and injections should be given, if necessary, based on the results of blood glucose checks.

*M*y doctor says we should induce
labor if it hasn't begun by
39–40 weeks. Why?

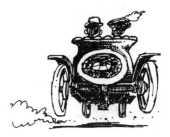

▼
TIP:

To ensure the safest delivery and the healthiest outcome for both you and your baby. Your health care team will determine the best time for delivery for you by considering your blood glucose control, blood pressure, kidney function, and any diabetes complication you may have. As you near the end of your pregnancy, your baby will also be evaluated for size, movement, heart rate, amniotic fluid, and lung maturity. Not too long ago, before more advanced fetal monitoring, diabetic pregnancies were induced a few weeks early to prevent large babies (sometimes called macrosomia) and late-term miscarriages. Now, with more advanced ways to manage your diabetes and your pregnancy, there is less need to induce pregnancies this early.

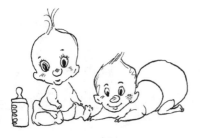

*W*ill *my baby's blood glucose levels be okay after delivery?*

▼
TIP:

This depends. Your blood glucose levels during pregnancy, labor, and delivery directly affect your baby's first blood glucose levels. If your blood glucose levels have been high throughout your pregnancy, your baby's pancreas will have been making extra insulin even before he or she is born. When delivered, your baby's glucose levels will drop dramatically from all of the extra insulin. This can lead to serious complications, such as seizures.

This rapid drop in blood glucose is common and your medical team will probably be prepared to check your baby's blood glucose levels as soon as he or she is delivered. If the baby's blood glucose is low, he or she will be given glucose in one form or another. Because this low blood sugar can stick around for 48 hours or may not even develop for 24 hours, your baby will be carefully watched, perhaps in a special care nursery.

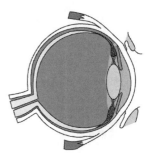

I have diabetic retinopathy. Will this be affected by the delivery of my baby?

▼
TIP:

Maybe, but there are ways to reduce your risk of worsening your retinopathy (complication of the eye). Good blood glucose control during pregnancy and laser photocoagulation treatments before pregnancy, if necessary, can go a long way toward lowering your risk. A baseline dilated eye exam is necessary before you become pregnant, and you should have your eyes checked regularly throughout your pregnancy. Still, your retinopathy may get worse during your pregnancy, especially if you have high blood glucose or high blood pressure.

Recent improvements in diabetes care have dramatically lowered the chances of complications for a mother during pregnancy. A complete evaluation by your medical team before pregnancy, along with an assessment of any complications you may have, can help a lot. And, as always, good blood glucose control is your best defense against complications.

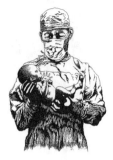

*W*hy *should a neonatologist be involved at my labor and delivery?*

▼
TIP:

Because if there are any problems at birth, a neonatologist can make sure your baby gets proper care. A neonatologist has special training in caring for babies that are sick and require intensive care after birth. They organize the care for your baby in the special care nursery or intensive care unit. Before your delivery, your obstetrician can talk with a neonatologist about the status of your diabetes, any pregnancies you have had before, and any complications you have had with this pregnancy. Using this information, a neonatologist can foresee any problems that may happen at delivery and afterward. More than likely, your delivery will go smoothly and your baby will be born without any problems. But having a neonatologist available will give you the security of knowing your baby will be handled by someone with special training, knowledge, and experience to handle any problems that may arise.

Chapter 10
AFTER YOUR BABY
IS BORN

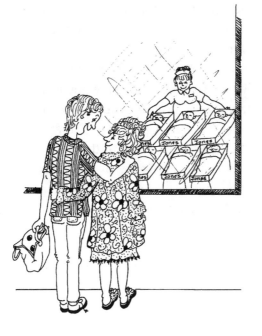

Since I had gestational diabetes, what are my chances of having diabetes later in life?

▼
TIP:

Higher than normal, but not certain. Although your glucose intolerance will probably disappear after your baby is born, the fact that you had gestational diabetes (GDM) does put you at a greater risk for developing type 2 later in life. In fact, 30–40% of women with GDM who are obese will develop type 2 diabetes within 4 years of their pregnancy. You can reduce your chances of developing type 2 diabetes by working to lose the weight you gained while you were pregnant. Exercise and physical activity are great ways to lose weight, plus it increases your sensitivity to insulin. There is also research that shows women with GDM who breastfeed have a lower rate of diabetes after pregnancy. Because you are at a higher risk for developing type 2 diabetes, you should be screened for diabetes every 3 years, at the minimum.

About 1/3 of women with a history of GDM also have high blood fat levels and an increased risk of heart disease. This is just another reason to eat healthy, control your weight, and get regular physical activity after your baby is born.

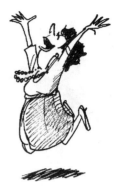

My gestational diabetes went away after my baby was born. Do I need to worry about it in future pregnancies?

▼
TIP:

Yes. If you've had gestational diabetes (GDM) before, you run a high risk of developing it again in future pregnancies, even though your blood glucose levels returned to normal after your baby was born. Your chances of developing GDM again are about 35–67%, although this can vary depending on risk factors, such as your ethnicity (higher in minority populations) and body weight (higher in obese women).

If you are planning another pregnancy, it is probably best that you be screened for diabetes before you become pregnant. Having high blood glucose levels when you conceive puts your baby at a higher risk for birth defects. If you've already become pregnant, you should be screened early in your pregnancy and again at 24–28 weeks if your early tests are negative. Staying lean and fit between pregnancies will lower your chances of developing diabetes in the future.

I had gestational diabetes. How soon after having the baby should I get my blood glucose rechecked?

▼
TIP:

About 6–8 weeks after delivery. Like 90% of the women with gestational diabetes (GDM), your blood glucose levels will probably return to normal right after your baby is born. However, you still run a very high risk of developing type 2 diabetes. In fact, 5% of women with GDM will have type 2 diabetes and 15% will have pre-diabetes by the time of this first screening. If your postpartum screening shows that you have pre-diabetes or glucose intolerance, you should seek advice on healthy eating, physical activity, and diabetes management. If your postpartum screening is negative, you should be retested every 3 years and before any future pregnancies.

C *an mothers with diabetes breastfeed*
their babies?

▼
TIP:

U nless your health care team advises you otherwise, yes. Breast milk provides the best nutrition for babies and breastfeeding is recommended for all mothers with either preexisting diabetes or gestational diabetes (GDM). Not only does breast milk have disease-fighting antibodies, it is also readily available, inexpensive, and convenient. There is also some evidence that breastfed babies may be protected from diabetes. And to top it all off, breastfeeding helps you lose weight!

Successful breastfeeding requires planning, mostly because breastfeeding causes your blood glucose levels to drop. You will need to pay close attention to your carbohydrate intake, physical activity, and insulin dosage (if necessary) while you are breastfeeding. If you are taking any oral medications to control your diabetes, ask your doctor whether or not they are safe to take while you are breastfeeding. If you have higher than normal blood glucose levels, you may be at risk for lactation-related infections, such as mastitis or thrush. For more information, you may want to talk with a lactation consultant (visit *www.ilca.org*) who is an expert in the art of breastfeeding for women with diabetes. Along with your friends, family, and health care team, this consultant can offer you the support you'll need to successfully breastfeed your baby.

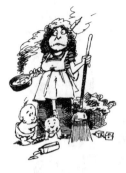

I would like to breastfeed my baby. Do I
need to make any changes to my diet?

▼
TIP:

Yes, a few subtle changes, but it's worth the extra effort. There
are many advantages to breastfeeding, especially excellent
nutrition for your developing child and some protection against
diabetes. Pay attention to your own nutrition as well. Making breast
milk requires extra calories, so you should probably add about
200 calories a day to the meal plan you were on while your were
pregnant. (Of course, burning those extra calories also helps you
lose weight.) Breastfeeding requires a lot of fluids, so be sure to get
plenty, at least 8–12 cups daily. You'll also need to pay close attention to your vitamin and mineral intake, especially calcium, zinc,
folate, and B vitamins. A prenatal vitamin supplement might help
ensure you're getting proper nutrition.

Breastfeeding will lower your blood glucose, putting you at an
increased risk of hypoglycemia (low blood glucose), especially if you
are taking insulin. Since most hypoglycemia occurs within an hour of
breastfeeding, it makes sense to work some snacks into your meal
plan. A good rule of thumb is to eat a snack when the baby is nursing,
particularly before bed and in the middle of the night. Your insulin
dose may need to be adjusted, so check your blood glucose often.

Once it is time to wean to your baby, you'll need to keep in
mind that your blood glucose levels will rise as you produce less
milk. During this period of adjustment, you'll probably want to cut
back on your calories and carbohydrates and check your blood
glucose more often. The weaning process should be gradual, lasting
2–3 months, with one feeding eliminated every week.

Will my insulin dose change now that I've had the baby?

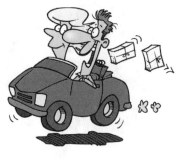

TIP:

Yes. While you are pregnant, contrainsulin hormones and weight gain make your body less sensitive to insulin. As a result, you require more insulin to keep your blood glucose under control. Once you deliver your baby, these contrainsulin hormones disappear. If you have type 1 or type 2 diabetes and take insulin, you may not need insulin for as long as 48–72 hours after the baby is born. Within a few weeks, your insulin needs will return to what they were before you were pregnant. Be sure to check your blood glucose frequently while you are making the adjustment back to your old insulin regimen.

If you have had gestational diabetes (GDM), your blood glucose will probably return to normal as soon as the baby is born. If you've been taking insulin during your pregnancy, you will probably no longer need to do so. However, you are at an increased risk of developing diabetes in the future, so you will need to be checked for glucose intolerance on a regular basis after your baby is born.

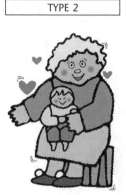

Now that I have had the baby, can I go back to taking the oral diabetes medications I took before I was pregnant?

▼

TIP:

Not right away. If you were taking oral medications before you were pregnant, and then switched to insulin during your pregnancy, you should probably stay on insulin for at least a month while your body adjusts to changing glucose levels. If you are breastfeeding, you also need to be sure your medications pose no risk to your baby. Tolbutamide is a blood glucose-lowering medication that is classified as a maternal medication and is usually OK to use while you're breastfeeding. However, there is little to no research on newer medications and their effects on breastfeeding. While it looks to be safe to breastfeed your child while using oral medications, you need to keep in mind that these medications can cross into breast milk. If you feel this is a problem, you should probably stick with insulin. Talk with your health care team about the best medication for you to take after your baby is born.

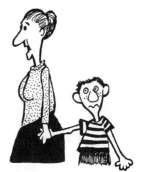

*W*ill my baby inherit diabetes from me?

▼
TIP:

This all depends on certain risk factors. The following chart shows the risks of your child developing diabetes based on family risk factors.

Family Member with Diabetes	Chance Child Will Develop Diabetes
No Diabetes in the Family	11% chance of type 2 diabetes by age 70 1% chance of type 1 diabetes by age 50
One Parent with Type 1 Diabetes Father with type 1 diabetes Mother with diabetes who was younger than 25 when the child was born Mother with diabetes who was older than 25 when the child was born	*(Risk doubles if the parent was diagnosed by the age of 11)* 6% chance of type 1 diabetes 4% chance of type 1 diabetes 1% chance of type 1 diabetes
One Parent with Type 2 Diabetes Diagnosed before the age of 50	14% chance of type 2 diabetes
Both Parents with Type 2 Diabetes Overall risk	45% chance of type 2 diabetes by age 65

In addition, gestational diabetes occurs more frequently in women who have a family history of diabetes.

Chapter 11
Preventing Pregnancy
Control Before Conception

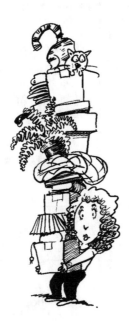

I *don't think I can get pregnant.*
Do I still need a contraceptive?

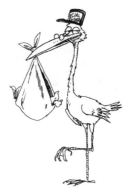

▼
TIP:

U nless you have a medical reason that absolutely confirms you cannot have a child (like a hysterectomy, for instance), you should use a contraceptive. Contraceptives are a vital part of good reproductive health for women during childbearing years, especially those with diabetes, since planning your pregnancy is very important. If you have high blood glucose at conception and through the first few weeks of your pregnancy, the chances of your child suffering birth defects are very high. Having your blood glucose under control *before* conception is an absolutely essential part of a pregnancy with diabetes. Even if you have only had gestational diabetes, prepregnancy planning is important, since you are at an increased risk of developing type 2 diabetes. Therefore, even though you don't *think* or *feel* that you can get pregnant, you should use a contraceptive throughout your childbearing years, which can last from puberty to menopause. Talk with your doctor about the types of contraceptives available and which one may be right for you.

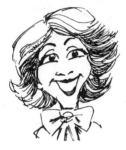

I've heard that women with diabetes can't take birth control pills. Is this true?

▼
TIP:

Not at all. Women with diabetes (or at risk for diabetes) can safely take birth control pills. While the use of any contraceptive should be discussed with your health care team to ensure that it will be safe and effective, contraceptive use in general is strongly recommended for women with diabetes to safeguard against unplanned pregnancies. The birth control pill seems to be especially effective in this regard. Plus, studies have shown that estrogen, which is in many oral contraceptives, has a positive effect on blood fat levels—it raises HDL, or "good cholesterol," and lowers LDL, or "bad cholesterol." However, the pill is not for everyone. If you are a smoker, have a heart condition, or suffer from complications of diabetes, such as retinopathy or nephropathy, the pill may not be right for you.

I don't want to take birth control pills.
What other contraceptives are there?
How well do they work?

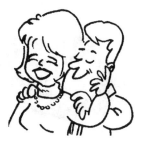

▼
TIP:

The following chart lists the types of contraceptive available,
their rate of effectiveness, and comments on each.

Type	Effectiveness	Comments
Oral Contraceptives Combined (*estrogen + progestin* or sequential)	98%	Associated with a variety of heart problems and complications. Still the pill of choice if estrogen is less than 35 mg.
Progestin only	94%	May increase serum lipids and glucose levels (may cause problems if you have a history of GDM)
Norplant System	99% (1st year) 96 % (yrs 2–5)	Menstrual irregularities

May increase serum lipids and increase glucose intolerance/insulin requirements.

Risk of infection at implant site |
Sterilization	99%	Cannot be reversed
Intrauterine Devices Progesterone containing	97%	May cause pain, irregular bleeding, perforation of uterus, infection, and possible increased failure rate
Copper device	97%	Does not need to be removed and reinserted every year
Diaphragm without Spermacide	82%	High failure rate
Condom + Foam	88%	High failure rate, but may prevent some sexually transmitted diseases
Contraceptive Sponge	72%	High failure rate
Cervical Cap	82%	Increased rate of abnormal pap smear
Rhythm Method	80%	Women with diabetes may have irregular periods, which increases the failure rate

Adapted from *Medical Management of Pregnancy Complicated by Diabetes*, 3rd ed., ADA, 2000.

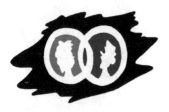

Can I get pregnant while taking the pill? If so, what do I do?

▼
TIP:

Yes, you can still get pregnant while taking the pill. Oral contraceptives are only 98% effective at best, which is a pretty good rate. However, some versions of the pill can become less effective if you don't take your doses within 24 hours of one another. Be sure you understand how you need to take your oral contraceptive, and what actions can make it less effective. Still, even if you take your pill exactly as prescribed, you could end up one of the 2% who becomes pregnant. If this happens, it's best to be prepared for pregnancy. Talk to your health care team as soon as possible. They can evaluate your health status and determine if there are any potential risks that may arise from the pregnancy. More than likely, your doctor will tell you to stop taking the pill right away. If necessary, you might talk to a behavior specialist who can help you pinpoint any emotional or psychological needs that may act as barriers to your mental and physical health.

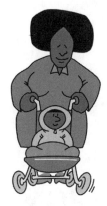

I didn't think you could get pregnant while breastfeeding. Can you?

▼
TIP:

Yes, you can. Breastfeeding is not a form of birth control. It is true that breastfeeding can have contraceptive effects if your baby is *exclusively* breastfed—no bottles or pacifiers at all—and you have not started menstruating for 6 months after you delivered the baby. But this is not reliable as a sole means of birth control. Talk with your doctor about which birth control methods would work best for you as a breastfeeding mother. Ask about how the method is used and how it will affect your blood glucose control, as well as any risks it may pose to you or your baby. But by all means, continue to breastfeed if you have your doctor's OK. Breastfeeding provides the ideal nutrition for your baby in the first 6 months of his or her life.

Chapter 12
PREGNANCY
POTPOURRI

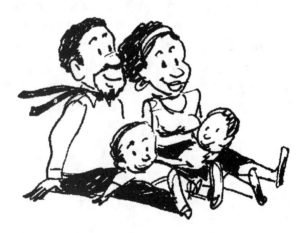

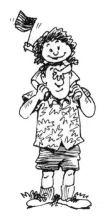

I have a family history of diabetes. What are my chances of developing diabetes while I am pregnant?

▼
TIP:

If you have a strong family history of type 2 diabetes, you run a much higher risk for developing gestational diabetes (GDM). Since you are at a higher risk, you should undergo blood glucose testing as early as possible during your pregnancy, ideally at your first prenatal visit. If your blood glucose levels are OK and there's no sign of gestational diabetes at this time, then you should be retested for GDM at 24–28 weeks of pregnancy. It is very, very important that you inform your health care professional of your medical history, including any family history of diabetes, especially in parents, siblings, and/or children with diabetes.

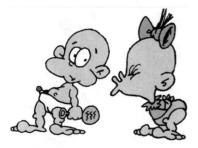

I have a sister who developed type 1 diabetes while she was pregnant. Will this happen to me?

▼
TIP:

Your sister's case is rare. Most often, if diabetes develops during pregnancy, it is referred to as gestational diabetes (GDM). GDM is defined as "any degree of glucose intolerance with onset or first recognition during pregnancy." This definition applies to any woman who develops diabetes during pregnancy, whether or not the diabetes continues once the baby is delivered. In most cases, GDM disappears after pregnancy. However, there are instances when the onset of type 1 or type 2 diabetes can actually occur at the same time as pregnancy. Pregnancy does not necessarily cause this to happen—it's just a coincidence. Your chances of developing type 1 diabetes are the same whether you are pregnant or not. Since your sister (a first-degree relative) developed type 1 diabetes, you are at a much higher risk for developing type 1 diabetes as well. There are tests that look for immune-related "markers," which can determine your likelihood of developing type 1 diabetes.

A bout 18 weeks into my pregnancy I noticed some dark skin around my neck. My doctor says I have insulin resistance. Does that mean I have diabetes?

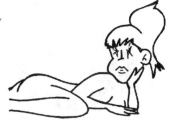

▼
TIP:

Not necessarily, but you may very well be on your way. The darkening around your neck is probably "acanthosis nigracans." Acanthosis nigracans is considered a sign of insulin resistance. Type 2 diabetes and gestational diabetes (GDM) are among several conditions associated with insulin resistance. If you are pregnant and have signs of insulin resistance, you should be considered a high risk for gestational diabetes and you should be screened for gestational diabetes as soon as possible. If your blood glucose levels are normal at the first screening, then you should be screened again at 24–28 weeks. As your pregnancy progresses, so does insulin resistance, especially around the 18–24th week. When this happens, your body probably won't be able to maintain good blood glucose control. At this point, GDM is usually diagnosed.

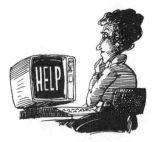

I did a search on the Internet for "diabetes and pregnancy" and thousands of resources came up. How do I know which ones might be useful?

▼
TIP:

The Internet is a great way to get lots of information easily and quickly. The problem is figuring out whether or not the information you are getting is reliable and accurate. With so much information available, it's hard to decide which advice to take! To find the best health information on the Internet, follow these tips:

- Determine who sponsors or owns the website you are browsing. If it is a commercial company (like a drug company, for instance), they may be trying to push a product and skew their information toward this product.
- Look for websites that list the credentials and affiliations of the people who provide the information for the site.
- Double-check the information with your health care team. Reliable sites back up their claims with references to peer-reviewed medical literature and established scientific findings, rather than testimonials.
- Note the date of the research or information posted on the site and when it was last updated. Credible websites are updated often to share the most current scientific advice.
- The American Diabetes Association website (*www.diabetes.org*) has a wealth of information that is always reliable and up to date.

Check for a seal of approval from a voluntary organization that requires quality guidelines, such as Health on the Net. In all cases, keep in mind that even reliable health information from the Internet should not replace the advice of your health care team!

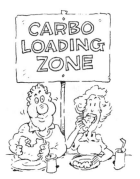

A week before I had my glucose
tolerance test, my doctor told me to
start eating a large breakfast of pancakes
with syrup before testing my blood
glucose levels. Why is this necessary?

▼
TIP:

B ecause pancakes and syrup are loaded with carbohydrates.
There are no specific foods that are *required* before your glucose tolerance test (GTT). The goal is simply to eat 150 grams or
more of carbohydrate each day *before* your test. (Most healthy
women, especially if they're pregnant, should consume at least this
much carbohydrate daily anyway.) Your doctor probably suggested
the pancakes and syrup as an example of carbohydrate-containing
foods to include during the 3-day period before your test. The
current American Diabetes Association recommendations prior to
the GTT procedure include:

- Eat "normally" for at least three days
- Unrestricted physical activity (within safe guidelines)
- No smoking the morning of or during the planned procedure
  (of course you shouldn't smoke at all, especially while you are
  pregnant!)
- Fasting at least 8 and no more than 14 hours before the GTT

It is usually best to schedule the GTT procedure first thing in the
morning, so you won't have to be without food all day.

Not all doctors suggest this carbohydrate increase before a GTT.
Some patients are confused by the seemingly mixed signals it gives
("Why does my doctor want me to eat this much carbohydrate if I
was just told I have diabetes?"). If you have any questions, be sure
to talk to your doctor.

INDEX

▼

A1C level, 4, 42, 61, 66
Alcohol, 33
Alpha-feta protein (AFP), 83
Amniocentesis, 21, 66
Artificial sweeteners, 31

Basal rate, 43
Birth defects, 2, 5, 12, 18, 33, 40, 61, 66, 82–83
Blood glucose screening, 10–11, 94, 109, 111
Body mass index (BMI), 23
Bolus amount, 43
Breastfeeding, 94, 97–98, 100, 107

Caffeine, 32
Carbohydrate, 26, 28–29, 31, 34–35, 56, 80, 113
Cesarean delivery, 57, 87
Complications, 2, 4, 6, 9, 44, 48, 55, 90–91
Constipation, 43
Contraception, 2, 7, 9, 103–107
Contrainsulin hormones, 15, 44, 63, 71, 76, 99

Dexamethasone, 21
Diabetes Food Pyramid, 26
Diabetes resources, 112

Edema, 81
Endocrinologist, 43, 66
Exercise, 7, 47–57, 76, 94, 113

Fish, 36
Fructosamine test, 67

Genetic counseling, 9
Glucagon, 19, 45
Glucose goals, 4, 60

Glucose intolerance, 29, 99
Glucose tolerance test GTT), 17, 113

Heart disease, 84, 94
Herbal remedies, 35
High blood sugar *See* Hypoglycemia
High blood pressure *See* Hypertension
High risk pregnancy, 6, 10, 12, 16, 25, 79, 81, 109–110
Hyperglycemia, 21, 40, 59, 80
Hypertension, 24, 81–82, 91
Hypoglycemia, 19–20, 35, 42, 45, 52, 59, 69, 98
Hypoglycemia unawareness, 19–20

Impaired glucose tolerance (IGT), 8
Insulin pump, 13, 40, 43, 88
Insulin regimen, 3, 20, 40–42, 44–45, 59, 62, 88, 99
Insulin resistance, 7–8, 44, 55, 111
Iron deficiency anemia, 12, 27

Ketoacidosis, 68
Ketones, 24, 30, 52, 68, 80
Ketonuria, 35

Labor & delivery, 87–92
Listeria monocytogenes, 37

Macrosomia, 40, 79, 89
Metformin, 7
Miscarriage, 5–6, 35, 39
Morning sickness, 35

Neonatologist, 66, 92
Nephropathy, 81
Nonstress Test (NST), 84
Nutritive sweeteners, 31

Obstetrician, 16, 21, 31–32, 44, 48, 64, 71, 87

Ophthalmologist, 85

Oral diabetes medications, 41, 44

Placenta crossing, 15, 25, 31–32, 44, 48, 64, 71, 87

Phenylketonuria, 21

Physical activity. *See* Exercise

Polycystic ovary syndrome (POS), 7

Postpartum depression, 57

Postpartum screening, 96

Pre-diabetes, 8

Preeclampsia, 24, 48

Prenatal vitamins, 12, 27

Prepregnancy planning, 3, 103

Registered Dietician (RD), 8, 28–30, 38, 80

Respiratory distress syndrome, 21

Retinopathy, 91

Risk factors, 101

Self monitoring, 28, 42, 57–67, 63–64, 69, 73, 75, 99

Smoking, 113

Snacks, 30, 35

Starvation ketosis, 30

Stress, 72–77, 80

Support groups, 74

Toxemia, 6, 81–82

Ultrasonography, 79

Walking, 49, 51, 53, 55–56, 77

Weight, 7, 10, 23, 25, 57, 62, 64, 80, 94–95

About the American Diabetes Association

The American Diabetes Association is the nation's leading voluntary health organization supporting diabetes research, information, and advocacy. Its mission is to prevent and cure diabetes and to improve the lives of all people affected by diabetes. The American Diabetes Association is the leading publisher of comprehensive diabetes information. Its huge library of practical and authoritative books for people with diabetes covers every aspect of self-care—cooking and nutrition, fitness, weight control, medications, complications, emotional issues, and general self-care.

To order American Diabetes Association books: Call 1-800-232-6733. http://store.diabetes.org [Note: there is no need to use **www** when typing this particular Web address]

To join the American Diabetes Association: Call 1-800-806-7801. www.diabetes.org/membership

For more information about diabetes or ADA programs and services: Call 1-800-342-2383. E-mail: Customerservice@diabetes.org www.diabetes.org

To locate an ADA/NCQA Recognized Provider of quality diabetes care in your area: www.ncqa.org/dprp/

To find an ADA Recognized Education Program in your area: Call 1-888-232-0822. www.diabetes.org/recognition/education.asp

To join the fight to increase funding for diabetes research, end discrimination, and improve insurance coverage: Call 1-800-342-2383. www.diabetes.org/advocacy

To find out how you can get involved with the programs in your community: Call 1-800-342-2383. See below for program Web addresses.

- *American Diabetes Month:* Educational activities aimed at those diagnosed with diabetes—month of November. www.diabetes.org/ADM
- *American Diabetes Alert:* Annual public awareness campaign to find the undiagnosed—held the fourth Tuesday in March. www.diabetes.org/alert
- *The Diabetes Assistance & Resources Program (DAR):* diabetes awareness program targeted to the Latino community. www.diabetes.org/DAR
- *African American Program:* diabetes awareness program targeted to the African American community. www.diabetes.org/africanamerican
- *Awakening the Spirit: Pathways to Diabetes Prevention & Control:* diabetes awareness program targeted to the Native American community. www.diabetes.org/awakening

To find out about an important research project regarding type 2 diabetes: www.diabetes.org/ada/research.asp

To obtain information on making a planned gift or charitable bequest: Call 1-888-700-7029. www.diabetes.org/ada/plan.asp

To make a donation or memorial contribution: Call 1-800-342-2383. www.diabetes.org/ada/cont.asp